OXFORD PSY

Depression in
Later Life

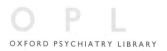

OXFORD PSYCHIATRY LIBRARY

Depression in Later Life

Robert C. Baldwin

Consultant Old Age Psychiatrist and
Honorary Professor of Psychiatry,
Manchester Mental Health and Social Care Trust,
Manchester Royal Infirmary,
Manchester, UK

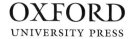

OXFORD
UNIVERSITY PRESS

OXFORD
UNIVERSITY PRESS

Great Clarendon Street, Oxford OX2 6DP

Oxford University Press is a department of the University of Oxford.
It furthers the University's objective of excellence in research, scholarship,
and education by publishing worldwide in

Oxford New York

Auckland Cape Town Dar es Salaam Hong Kong Karachi
Kuala Lumpur Madrid Melbourne Mexico City Nairobi
New Delhi Shanghai Taipei Toronto

With offices in

Argentina Austria Brazil Chile Czech Republic France Greece
Guatemala Hungary Italy Japan Poland Portugal Singapore
South Korea Switzerland Thailand Turkey Ukraine Vietnam

British Library Cataloguing in Publication Data

Data available

Library of Congress Cataloging in Publication Data

Data available

Typeset
Printed in
on acid-fr
L.E.G.O.

ISBN 978

10 9 8 7

Contents

Preface

As a specialty, old age psychiatry arose from the unique needs of old people with psychiatric disorder and the special knowledge and skills required to address these needs. The early pioneers had demonstrated that late-life mental disorders were not, as thought, simply an undifferentiated group of problems arising from 'senility' but could be clearly differentiated into distinct disorders with different prognoses. This, and the advent of antidepressants, led to a new optimism in treating mood disorders in later life. At the time I entered the field some 25 years ago, it was still relatively new. During this time I have witnessed an explosion of research into late-life depression which underpins the evidence base we now use to treat it and which I have tried to summarise in this book. The aim is to provide a resource to practitioners of different backgrounds who find themselves involved in the care of older people with depressive disorder.

Robert Baldwin
Manchester June 2009

Symbols and abbreviations

5-HT	5-hydroxytryptamine
APOE	apolipoprotein E
CBT	cognitive behavioural therapy
CHD	coronary heart disease
COPD	chronic obstructive pulmonary disease
CRF	corticotropin-releasing factor
CRH	corticotropin-releasing hormone
CT	computerized tomography
DEDS	depression-executive dysfunction syndrome
DSM	Diagnostic and Statistical Manual
ECA	epidemiologic catchment area
ECG	electrocardiogram
ECT	electroconvulsive therapy
EEG	electroencephalogram
FSC	front-striatal circuits
GDS	geriatric depression scale
GP	general practitioner
HADS	Hospital Anxiety and Depression Scale
HDRS	Hamilton depression rating scale
HPA	hypothalamic-pituitary-adrenal
IADH	inappropriate antidiuretic hormone
ICD	International Classification of Diseases
IPT	interpersonal therapy
MADRAS	Montgomery–Åsberg depression rating scale
MAOI	monoamine oxidase inhibitor
MMSE	mini-mental state examination
MRI	magnetic resonance imaging
NARI	noradrenaline (norepinephrine) reuptake inhibitor

NaSSA	noradrenergic and specific serotonergic antidepressant
NSAIDS	non-steroidal anti-inflammatory drugs
OMC	orientation memory-concentration
PET	positron emission tomography
PHQ	patient health questionnaire
PST	problem solving treatment
QoF	quality and outcomes framework
RCT	randomized controlled trial
RIMA	reversible inhibitors of monoamine oxidase A
rTMS	repetitive transcranial magnetic stimulation
SADQ-H	stroke aphasic depression questionnaire hospital version
SNRI	serotonin/noradrenaline reuptake inhibitor
SPECT	single photon emission computerized tomography
SSRI	selective serotonin reuptake inhibitor
TCA	tricyclic antidepressant
WML	white matter lesions

Chapter 1

Introduction

Lilly is 88 and her daily requests to be taken to see a doctor about her 'stomach wind' are wearing out her 60-year-old recently retired son, who is finding himself waking early in the morning with worry. John is 72 and devastated at the unexpected loss of his wife just before their fiftieth wedding anniversary. His family and friends are sympathetic but even after 6 months he is fretful, miserable, and feels he will burden people by talking about it. Wong-Chai has had arthritis for the past 20 of her 75 years. Once proud and indomitable she has lately found her joint pain unbearable and has wondered about 'going to sleep and never waking up'. Raj is 85 and lately finds himself unable to concentrate, to the extent that he keeps losing things. His sleep and appetite are poor and he has stopped going to the local day care centre. His doctor said it is his age but his family fear the start of dementia. Jack, aged 76, has turned up in the Emergency Department feeling nauseous and dizzy. Recently, he has lost weight and feels very tired, lonely, and miserable. He admits to taking four sleeping tablets last night 'just to get a bit of peace for the night'. The doctor tells him not to worry and that dose will not harm him. A week later he is back with a serious paracetamol overdose.

What links these vignettes is depressive disorder. Although dementia is regarded as the typical mental health complaint of later life, depression is far more common. Often overlooked, depression is a very serious problem in later life. It reduces the quality of life and adds to the disability associated with all the major medical illnesses that afflict older people. It not only complicates the course of dementia but also is a risk factor for it.

Epitomized by the statement 'who would not be depressed at that age?', it is tempting but completely inaccurate to assume that depression must be the norm in later life. In the main, health professionals see older people who are most susceptible to depression, those with frailty, and chronic medical illnesses. The trap then is to 'normalize' depression in older people who are ill with the result that major depression can be overlooked. In reality, many older people live contentedly with their quality of life improving with age (Netuveli et al. 2006). Among those who do become depressed, many have a definite mental health disorder and there are interventions which can help significantly.

There are already textbooks on depression, why then is one needed specifically for depression in later life? First, there is the self-evident fact that the world's population is fast growing older. This brings with it increasing rates of many of the common health problems, including depression. Second, although depression in later life shares many of the core features with depression at other times, there are some important differences. Third, late-life depression frequently occurs in the setting of significant medical morbidity which complicates both the diagnosis and the treatment. Finally, depression in this age group often presents with altered cognition, unravelling moods, and loss of memory.

This book sets out the core knowledge about late-life depressive disorders and summarizes the key evidence base for successful interventions relevant to practitioners who work with older people.

Key references

Netuveli G, Wiggins RD, Hildon Z, Montgomery SM, Blane D (2006). Quality of life at older ages: evidence from the English longitudinal study of aging (wave 1). *Journal of Epidemiology and Community Health*, **60**, 357–63.

Chapter 2

Classification and epidemiology

2.1 Types of depression in later life

Depression can mean a symptom or a syndrome. As a *symptom*, the key to distinguish morbid depression from the transitory low mood experienced by everyone from time to time is that in depression there is a qualitative change in mood. Those affected recognize these changes in mood themselves. They may also be aware that the duration and frequency differ (most days, most of the time) from transient unhappiness, and even positive events produce little relief.

In recent years, there has been a significant change in the way depression is conceptualized. Rather than fixed categories of depression into which the patient must be squeezed, the evidence suggests that depression is on a continuum from normal sadness to pathologically severe depression (Paykel and Priest 1992). Nevertheless, in psychiatry, as in the rest of medicine, practice would be impossible without some kind of classification and the most common approach is to set a threshold of symptoms above which a patient is said to have the *syndrome* of depression (Box 2.1). The threshold is set by criteria agreed via one of the two international systems of classification, the International Classification of Diseases (ICD-10) (World Health Organization

Box 2.1 DSM-IV criteria for major depressive disorder

(A) Five or more of the following symptoms should be present during the same 2-week period and represent change from previous functioning; at least one of the symptoms should be either (1) depressed mood or (2) loss of interest or pleasure.

Note: Symptoms that are clearly due to a general medical condition are not included.

(1) Depressed mood most of the day, nearly every day, as indicated by either subjective report (e.g., feels sad or empty) or observation made by others (e.g., appears tearful)

(2) Markedly diminished interest or pleasure in all, or almost all, activities most of the day (as indicated by either subjective account or observation made by others)

(3) Significant weight loss when not dieting or weight gain (e.g., a change of more than 5% of body weight in a month), or decrease or increase in appetite nearly every day

(4) Insomnia or hypersomnia nearly every day

(5) Psychomotor agitation or retardation nearly every day (observable by others, not merely subjective feelings of restlessness or being slowed down)

(6) Fatigue or loss of energy nearly every day

(7) Feelings of worthlessness or excessive or inappropriate guilt (which may be delusional) nearly every day (not merely self-reproach or guilt about being sick)

(8) Diminished ability to think or concentrate or indecisiveness, nearly every day (either by subjective account or as observed by others)

(9) Recurrent thoughts of death (not just fear of dying), recurrent suicidal ideation without a specific plan, or a suicide attempt or a specific plan for committing suicide.

(B) The symptoms do not meet the criteria for a Mixed Episode (of anxiety and depression).

(C) The symptoms cause clinically significant distress or impairment in social, occupational, or other important areas of functioning.

(D) The symptoms are not due to the direct physiological effects of a substance (e.g., a drug of abuse, a medication) or a general medical condition (e.g., hypothyroidism).

(E) The symptoms are not better accounted for by bereavement, i.e., after the loss of a loved one, the symptoms persist for longer than 2 months or are characterized by marked functional impairment, morbid preoccupations with worthlessness, suicidal ideation, psychotic symptoms, or psychomotor retardation.

Note: Specifiers can be coded for *severity* (mild, moderate, or severe), *psychosis* (mood-congruent or mood-incongruent delusions or hallucinations), and *remission* (partial or full).

1994) or the Diagnostic and Statistical Manual (DSM-IV) (American Psychiatric Association 1994). Although broadly similar, the latter is simpler to grasp and, according to evidences from research, more efficient in treatment. The DSM-IV scheme is outlined in Box 2.1 and specifies that five core symptoms must be present; at least one of the symptoms must be depressed mood or loss of interest or pleasure.

These symptoms must be present for at least 2 weeks and must be 'pervasive', that is, the symptoms must be there for most days, most of the time and must interfere with the way the person lives his/her life.

Patients with the syndrome of mild depressive disorder are distressed by their symptoms but can continue to function in life relatively normally. In moderate depression, the individual is more subjectively distressed and can maintain function but with considerable difficulty. Those with severe depression are generally in marked distress and are often agitated or retarded. The ability to function in usual roles is severely limited.

Just because a patient does not meet the diagnostic threshold it does not mean that their symptoms are unimportant. Having a few symptoms persistently, especially if accompanied by impaired function or quality of life, is a key risk factor for major depression. Often termed sub-threshold depression or minor depression (or dysthymia if chronic), this low-level depression is not trivial among the older population and is associated with adverse health effects, as discussed in the next section. Because sub-syndromal depression in later life is much more common than syndromal depression, its negative impact on the heath of the older population is greater.

To summarize, depressive disorder is the overall term for any form of depression likely to require or benefit from intervention. The two main categories of depressive disorder are major depression and sub-threshold (sub-syndromal) depression. Table 2.1 incorporates some of the other terms that may be encountered and gives the relevant codes from the two major international classificatory systems discussed earlier (Anderson *et al.* 2008). ICD-10 and DSM-IV differ slightly in that in ICD-10 only four symptoms are needed to make a diagnosis of depressive episode; this milder form of depression is included under sub-threshold depression.

2.1.1 Differential diagnosis

The conditions to consider when interviewing a patient with significant depressive symptoms are shown in Box 2.2.

Depressive disorder is termed 'organic' if there is evidence of a direct link between the onset of depression and either a systemic or neurological condition or an ingested substance or drug. Causes are discussed in more detail in Chapter 5. Depression accompanying dementia may be classified here; but in DSM-IV, depression with dementia is separately classified. Do not forget that alcohol can precipitate or prolong depression.

Table 2.1 Classifying depressive disorder

Classification used in this book	DSM-IV (code)	ICD-10 (code)
Major depression	Major depressive episode, single episode or recurrent (296)	Depressive episode severe (F32.2), moderate (F32.1), or mild with at least five symptoms (F32.0) Recurrent depressive disorder current episode severe (F33.2), moderate (F33.1), or mild with at least five symptoms (F33.0)
Sub-threshold depression (includes 'minor' depression)	Depressive disorder not otherwise specified (311)	Depressive episode, mild with four symptoms (F32.0) Recurrent depressive disorder current episode mild with four symptoms (F33.0) Mixed anxiety and depressive disorder (F41.2)
	Adjustment disorder with depressed mood/mixed anxiety and depressed mood (309)	Adjustment disorder—depressive reaction/mixed anxiety and depressive reaction (F43.2) Other mood (affective) disorders (F38)
	Dysthymia (300.4)	Dysthymia (F34.1)

Box 2.2 Differential diagnoses of depression

Major depressive disorder
Organic depressive disorder
Bipolar affective disorder
Psychotic depression
Dysthymia
Mixed anxiety and depression
Adjustment disorder

Bipolar disorder with an onset in later life is infrequent but recurrent bipolar disorder (earlier in adulthood) causing bouts of depression is not uncommon. This is known as 'bipolar depression'.

Dysthymia is a chronic depression with duration of at least 2 years and a number of symptoms from Box 2.1, although less than that required for major depression. It is often difficult to separate this concept from depressive personality traits or, in older people, the depleting emotional effects of living with chronic handicapping illness.

In mixed anxiety and depressive disorder, symptoms of depression and anxiety are both present but below the threshold for either depressive episode or generalized anxiety disorder. Finally, adjustment disorder with depressive reaction is diagnosed when depressive symptoms below the threshold for a diagnosis of depressive episode begin within a month of a serious threat or loss. Symptoms usually resolve within 6 months.

Psychosis can lead to depressive symptoms. Usually, it is clear that the patient's major problem is the presence of delusions and/or hallucinations. By convention in psychotic conditions mild to moderate depressive symptoms are considered as secondary to psychosis. A severely depressed patient may present with psychotic symptoms. If due to depression, psychotic experiences are usually 'congruent' with the mood, then the mood is related to depressive themes of low self-esteem or hopelessness. Occasionally, this is not the case—psychotic symptoms are non-congruent—in which case the relative importance of the two sets of symptoms, depression and psychosis, must be weighed up. The particular problem of hypochondriacal delusions is discussed in a later section.

2.2 Epidemiology

At all ages, the prevalence of sub-threshold depression significantly exceeds that of major depression. Early research (Kay et al. 1964) found that 10% of older adults in the community had what would now correspond to sub-threshold depression (i.e., significant symptoms but below the threshold for major depression), but only 1.3% met criteria for what we now call major depression. Remarkably, similar figures were found in the much more recent EURO-DEP study of depression in later life conducted in 14 countries—between 8.6% and 14.1% for depressive disorder overall and 1%–4% for major depression (Copeland et al. 1999).

The above rates of major depression are lower than those for younger adults. A low rate was also found in the influential North American Epidemiologic Catchment Area (ECA) study (Blazer 2003). Several explanations for the age-related differences in prevalence have been proposed. First, for reasons we do not know, the prevalence of major depression may fall with age. Second, the rates may be underestimates because studies often exclude individuals in care homes, where the prevalence of depression is high. Excluding people with depressive symptoms soon after bereavement from being diagnosed with depressive disorder is likely to disproportionately affect rates of diagnosis in older people—until recently this was the convention (Box 2.1). Third, the strict checklist approach of DSM and ICD to diagnosing major depression may not be suited to older populations. There is some evidence for this. Prince *et al.* (1999) used an age-specific depression scale, 'EURO-D', to compare symptoms of depression among older adults in Europe. Two factors encapsulated the majority of depressive symptoms. One factor was 'affective suffering' (characterized by depression, tearfulness, and a wish to die) and the other factor was a 'motivation' factor (comprising loss of interest, poor concentration, and lack of enjoyment). It was the motivation factor that tends to increase with age rather than affective suffering, which remained constant across age groups. This constellation of symptoms does not lend itself readily to ICD-10 and DSM-IV, so it is likely that the prevalence of depressive disorder does not appreciably fall with age and may even increase when co-morbidity from depleting medical conditions are factored in.

Medical co-morbidity and cognitive impairment are the two key factors that affect the diagnosis and management of depressive disorder in older adults. Because of this, rates of depression (including major depression) in long-term care facilities such as residential and nursing homes are typically up to three times higher than among community residents (Blazer 2003). The combination of physical frailty and cognitive impairment results in even higher rates.

A similar picture is seen among older patients admitted to the medical and surgical wards of acute hospitals with figures averaging 10%–12% for major depression (Blazer 2003). Cognitive impairment is also associated with high rates of depression, with rates of 17% for Alzheimer's disease and even higher for vascular and sub-cortical dementias (Alexopoulos 2005).

Is age itself a risk factor for depression? In a large cohort study, Robert *et al.* (1997) found that *healthy* older people were not at greater risk of depression than younger ones. Higher prevalence with age was explained by the poorer health of the older subjects rather than their age.

2.3 Impact of depression

By the year 2020, the World Health Organization predicts that depression will be the leading illness associated with negative impact and disease burden on human well-being, replacing communicable diseases and overtaking other conditions such as ischaemic heart disease, neoplastic diseases, and cerebrovascular disease. Latest estimates from the Global Burden of Disease study (GBD 2000) indicated that unipolar depressive disorders accounted for 4.4% of the global disease burden (65 million disability adjusted life years [DALYs] lost in total), in the same range as the total burden attributable to ischaemic heart disease, diarrhoeal diseases, or the combined impact of asthma and chronic obstructive pulmonary disease (World Health Organization 2002).

Sub-threshold depression is associated with functional impairment approaching that of major depression (Blazer 2003). Risk factors for sub-threshold depression (minor depression) in later life are similar to those for major depression. Minor (sub-threshold) depression is also a risk factor for major depressive episode. Given the scale of sub-threshold depression it alone adds substantially to the burden due to depression.

Key references

Alexopoulos GS (2005). Depression in the elderly. *The Lancet*, **365**(9475), 1961–70.

American Psychiatric Association (1994). *Diagnostic and statistical manual version IV*. APA, Washington DC.

Anderson IM, Ferrier IN, Baldwin R, *et al.* (2008). On behalf of the consensus meeting; endorsed by the British Association for Psychopharmacology. Evidence-based guidelines for treating depressive disorders with antidepressants: a revision of the 2000 British Association for Psychopharmacology guidelines. *Journal of Psychopharmacology*, **22**, 343–96.

Blazer DG (2003). Depression in late life: review and commentary. *Journal of Gerontology: Medical Sciences*, **58A**, 249–65.

Copeland JRM, Beekman ATF, Dewey ME, *et al.* (1999). Depression in Europe: geographical distribution among older people. *British Journal of Psychiatry*, **174**, 312–21.

Kay DW, Beamish P, and Roth M (1964). Old age mental disorders in Newcastle Upon Tyne, Part I: a study of prevalence. *British Journal of Psychiatry*, **110**, 146–58.

Paykel ES and Priest RG (1992). Recognition and management of depression in general practice: consensus statement. *British Medical Journal*, **305**, 1198–202.

Prince MJ, Beekman ATF, Deeg DJH, *et al.* (1999). Depression symptoms in late life assessed using the EURO-D scale: effect of age, gender and marital status in 14 European centers. *British Journal of Psychiatry*, **174**(4), 339–45.

Robert RE, Kaplan GA, Shema SJ, Strawbridge WJ (1997). Does growing old increase the risk for depression? *American Journal of Psychiatry*, **154**, 1384–90.

World Health Organization (1994). *The ICD-10 classification of mental and behavioural disorders*. WHO, Geneva.

World Health Organization (2002). The World Health Report 2002; reducing risks. Promoting health life. WHO, Geneva.

Chapter 3

Clinical features

> **Key points**
> - Two main differences in the presentation of late-life depression are that a complaint of depression may be minimized and somatic concern (hypochondriasis) is present.
> - Apathy and depression differ and the former is often associated with executive cognitive problems and vascular brain disease.
> - Attempted suicide in older adults closely resembles successful suicide.
> - Cognitive impairment is common in late-life depression and is often irreversible.

3.1 Symptoms

3.1.1 Key age-related factors

Brodaty *et al.* (2001) examined the effect of age of onset on the phenomenology of late-life depression in 810 patients referred to a tertiary mood disorders service in Australia. Some clinical types, such as psychotic depression, and some clinical features, such as psycho-motor agitation or retardation, marked withdrawal, hypochondriasis, and severe guilt, were more common in older patients and were associated more with age than with age at onset, an effect more pronounced in females. In this study, subjective reports of depressed mood were lower in older patients whereas objective measures were higher. This disparity increased markedly with age and supports the view that older patients minimize feelings of sadness.

Taken together, data like these suggest that there are two key features that distinguish late-life depressive disorders in older people: when depressed they complain less of sadness than younger adults and they often become excessively concerned about physical health (somatic concern or hypochondriasis). Depression without sadness is not the contradiction that it sounds because on more detailed inter-view there will invariably be other symptoms of depressive disorder (Box 2.1); the problem is that these two key features can obscure the diagnosis of depression.

Why these changes in the presentation of depression in later life occur is a matter of speculation but generational differences probably play a large part. Those who grew up after the austerity which followed the First World War learned to be stoic and to 'not bother the doctor' with emotional difficulties. As children, strict toilet training and the observance of a regular bowel habit were probably more ingrained which might explain why the bowel becomes such a frequent preoccupation among older people when depressed.

A point to be aware of is that there is sometimes a 'disconnect' between the older people's medical history and their hypochondriacal complaints when depressed. For example, a patient may have good reasons to be concerned about their heart if they suffer from ischaemic heart disease causing breathlessness and angina. When depressed he or she may present with heightened anxiety and preoccupation about the heart but, for reasons we cannot explain, in another scenario the person may present with quite unrelated concerns; for example, fear of bowel blockage. This can lead to two mistakes. The practitioner may go on a 'wild goose chase' looking for evidence of a worsened cardiac state in the first scenario, overlooking the depressive disorder causing the increased cardiac concern. Equally in the second scenario, speculative investigations may be undertaken in an attempt to link known pathology to the new presentation; again missing the depression. However, there is a need to conduct appropriate investigation of newly presenting depressive disorder and this will be considered in Chapter 6.

3.1.2 Psychosis

Although there is some debate as to whether psychotic (delusional) symptoms in depression simply reflect a more severe form of depression or represent a specific subtype, there does seem to be a higher likelihood of this occurring in late-life depression. The classical delusions of depression include guilt, poverty, and worthlessness, but in older age hypochondriacal delusions are often prominent (Baldwin 1995). Another psychotic presentation is Cotard's syndrome, where patients may negate their own body or their existence. For example, a severely depressed patient once dismissed the author by saying that there was no point in any questions as she was already dead and was awaiting the ambulance to take her body away. Abnormal perceptions, such as auditory hallucinations, may also occur in severe depression. Usually, these take the form of a voice in the second person making derogatory remarks. The content is often 'congruent' with the mood (e.g. 'you're worthless' in someone with very negative views of self). Box 3.1 illustrates some vignettes.

A 75-year-old man was admitted to the hospital after cutting his wrist. He was clearly depressed but after 6 weeks treatment with an antidepressant there was little improvement. His lack of reassurance about his health (which was good), increasing requests to see 'the chief doctor', and the uncovering of an earlier history of profound weight loss eventually diagnosed as depression made the treating team suspect delusions. Eventually, he confessed to an unshakeable belief that he had syphilis. A negative test briefly reassured him, but his delusion only left after introducing an antipsychotic drug. The final diagnosis was psychotic depression.

An 86-year-old woman of anxious disposition presented to her primary care physician 3 weeks after seeing her hairdresser whom she believed may have accidentally introduced 'some sort of infection' via hair curlers. Despite reassurance, she presented serially with complaints that her scalp was itchy and that her cheeks were 'on fire' preventing her from sleeping. Realizing that this must be a psychological complaint, the physician uncovered low mood, marked morning anxiety, early morning waking, and decreased function. Moderate non-psychotic depressive disorder diagnosed was caused by recent worries about her husband's ill-health.

Sometimes detecting psychotic beliefs can be difficult in profoundly withdrawn patients. It is one of the factors to consider in patients with treatment-resistant depression, as depression with psychotic symptoms rarely responds to an antidepressant alone. This is discussed further in Chapter 6 but clues include a past history of this presentation (as psychosis in depression tends to 'run true'), frequent muttering or distraction as if responding to internal or external stimuli, oppositional behaviour suggesting persecutory ideation (e.g., believing food is poisoned), and escalating requests for medical help regarding specific symptoms that have already been addressed.

3.1.3 Apathy and amotivation

Apathy (literally a loss of 'pathos') is generally defined as a lack of goal-directed activity or thought and/or a lack of goal-related emotional response. Often it is summarized as 'the spark is missing' (Van Reekum *et al.* 2005). As a disorder of motivation rather than mood, apathy is distinct from depression. Similar to depression, apathy is used to denote either a symptom or a syndrome. The syndromal aspects may be experienced in the affective, behavioural, or cognitive domains, resulting in indifference, indolence, and impoverished thoughts, respectively. It is associated with stroke, traumatic brain injury, frontal lobe degeneration, degenerative dementias, multiple sclerosis, and depressive disorder (Van Reekum *et al.* 2005). It is particularly seen in basal ganglia diseases and conditions that disrupt the integrity of the subcortical–frontal connections, especially involving the anterior cingulate and the dorsolateral prefrontal cortex. Together these are known as front-striatal circuits (FSCs). FSCs are important in late-life depression as any disruption causes a 'dysexecutive syndrome', a cognitive syndrome that will be discussed in the next section.

Apathy is not the same as depression although there is overlap. How can the two be distinguished? As shown in Figure 3.1, depressive disorder is a disorder of mood which often has secondary effects on motivation and is experienced as highly distressing for the individual. Apathy is primarily a disorder of motivation that decreases subjective response, including distress, which is therefore felt more by caregivers. Box 3.2 offers a vignette. Depression responds to psychological treatments and medication whilst apathy may require a behavioural intervention.

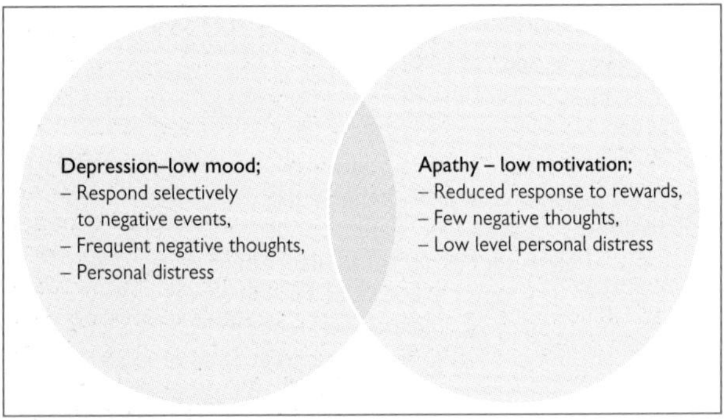

14

Depression–low mood;
– Respond selectively
   to negative events,
– Frequent negative thoughts,
– Personal distress

Apathy – low motivation;
– Reduced response to rewards,
– Few negative thoughts,
– Low level personal distress

Figure 3.1 The overlap between depression and apathy.

Box 3.2 Vignette: apathy and depression

A 68-year-old man presented with food refusal and 15kg weight loss. His wife had died a year earlier, and impaired mobility had led to the admission to a nursing home during which time the weight loss had occurred. Staff brought food to his room but were usually dismissed with a curt remark about not being bothered with food, although sometimes if they left food it would be eaten. Lately, instead of merely declining food he became hostile and swore; his sleep was disrupted and he reported having a lot more back pain. He was admitted to the psychiatric unit where moderate depressive disorder was diagnosed and investigations revealed multiple degenerative vertebral disc fractures. Treatment comprised an antidepressant and revision of analgesia. His mood and irritability improved but his apathy regarding food required the introduction of a structured behavioural programme aimed at reinforcing pleasurable aspects of eating and discouraging eating alone in his room. With this his weight increased.

3.1.4 **Typical presentations**

Although there are few symptoms which incontrovertibly distinguish late-life from early-onset depression, there are differences in clinical presentation. As discussed, a complaint of depression is understated among older people and may be attributed to physical illness, although there is of course a significant overlap of depressive symptoms and physical illness. These considerations may accentuate some aspects of presentation whilst other factors tend to obscure the diagnosis (Box 3.3).

A frequent difficulty is the overlap of depression with co-morbid medical illness. DSM-IV takes an aetiological approach to mood symptoms, meaning that the clinician must judge whether a symptom (e.g., reduced appetite) is due to physical illness and if so discount it in diagnosing depression. The opposite, the inclusive approach, is to make no aetiological assumptions and count all symptoms, whether or not better explained by co-morbid illnesses. Koenig *et al.* (1997) applied a range of strategies from the purely aetiological approach to an inclusive one and showed, not surprisingly, that they resulted in a twofold difference in the assessed prevalence of major depression.

Take the following example. An individual with active rheumatoid arthritis may experience insomnia, fatigue, and poor appetite equally from his or her physical illness or an associated depression. For a practitioner with little experience in mental health, the inclusive approach will probably be the safest but may result in overdiagnosing depression. A more experienced person will want to make a judgement about the likelihood of this symptom being more likely to be due to depression or medical co-morbidity. The history is key.

Box 3.3 Important aspects of the clinical presentation of late-life depression

- Minimal expression of sadness
- Somatization or excessive physical (hypochondriacal) complaints
- Overlap of physical and somatic psychiatric symptoms
- Unexplained pain syndromes
- Neurotic symptoms of recent onset
- Medically 'trivial' acts of deliberate self-harm
- 'Pseudodementia'
- Depression superimposed upon dementia
- Accentuation of abnormal personality traits
- Behaviour disorder
- Late-onset alcohol dependency syndrome
- 'Loneliness'
- Insomnia

For example, early morning wakening may emerge from a background of more generalized sleep disturbance due to pain. Questions must be appropriate. For example, for those with limited mobility or exercise tolerance a question such as 'Do you feel tired even when resting?' is preferable to 'Have you no energy?'. With the patient's permission, a history from someone close is often informative as is uncovering prior episodes of depression, which may provide a pointer to the current disorder.

There is growing awareness that depression may present predominantly with pain. The pain is often non-specific. Headache, abdominal pain, or musculoskeletal pains in the lower back, joints, and neck are common and may occur in combination so that the clinician should have a high index of suspicion in patients presenting with multiple pain symptoms of unclear aetiology.

So-called neurotic symptoms of recent onset in later life should not be taken at face value. The sudden occurrence of marked anxiety, obsessional compulsive phenomena, hysteria, or hypochondriasis in an older person not previously neurotically prone should serve as a prompt to look closely for depressive disorder, which is the usual cause. Likewise, at all levels of severity of depression, anxiety is a common accompanying symptom. If it dominates the clinical picture it may mask the depressive disorder.

'Pseudodementia' has been used in several different ways but most characteristically when an older patient presents with vociferous complaints of poor memory, many 'don't know' responses, and a relatively recent onset. Although these patients appear to be amnesic with poor attention, they do not have deficits in higher cortical function, such as aphasia, agraphia, or acalculia, which suggest an underlying dementia. Pseudodementia is a term which has probably outlived its usefulness. Other terms such as 'Dementia of Depression' (Pearlson et al. 1989) and 'Depression–Executive Dysfunction Syndrome (DEDS)' (Alexopoulos et al. 2002) are now used (see Section 3.3).

Less discussed in the literature but readily recognizable to clinicians working with older patients is when depression shows itself under the guise of a disorder of behaviour. Presentations with food refusal, 'incontinence' (e.g., a perverse ability to eliminate in almost any place other than the toilet, unlike the incontinence of dementia), screaming, and outwardly aggressive behaviour may occur, often in a residential or nursing home facility where the person is resentful of having been admitted. A history from someone who knows the patient is crucial. This will often highlight a recent change in mood and vitality.

The advent of depressive disorder may lead to a dramatic accentuation in pre-morbid personality. A previously anxious and dependent person when depressed may present with theatricality and ceaseless importuning, sometimes to several agencies simultaneously; for example, social services, primary care, and the local Accident and Emergency Department. Other behavioural problems that may occur indicate underlying depressive disorder in older people, which include shoplifting in a hitherto honest person and late-onset alcohol dependence syndrome.

A complaint of loneliness from an individual, who previously coped quite well alone, often accompanied by a request to be rehoused, should raise a suspicion of depressive disorder.

There is a complex relationship between insomnia and depression. It is both a symptom which heralds depression and a risk factor for it. Because insomnia occurs more frequently with age, it can too readily be dismissed as 'ageing'. It is a serious symptom of depression, can be one of the last to resolve with treatment, and contributes to the risk of suicide in major depression.

3.2 Suicide (see also Sections 7.3 and 8.4)

Attempted suicide in older adults closely resembles successful suicide in its clinical characteristics. A (literally) fatal mistake then is not to take seriously an act of deliberate self-harm because it appears to be medically trivial. Elderly people rarely take overdoses merely to draw attention, to resolve tension, or merely by accident. Most have depressive disorder and all require a psychiatric assessment. More difficult to characterize is the concept of depression presenting as 'sub-intentional' suicide. This might be suspected in individuals who are profoundly withdrawn, reject assistance, refuse food, and suffer severe weight loss. However, patients who 'turn their face to the wall' are a heterogeneous group, some of whom may be severely depressed but others turn out to have hidden medical problems such as carcinoma.

It is clearly important to recognize older people at risk of suicide. Previous self-harm is the factor most predictive of suicide. Several other factors add to the risk. Box 3.4 lists them under three headings: general factors in the community, features of depression, and specific behaviours. The means of suicide in older people vary from culture to culture. Overdose, especially of benzodiazepines and non-opiate analgesics, is common in Western cultures; however in the United States, firearm use by older men is becoming more frequent.

Box 3.4 Suicide risk in later life

General factors

Any past suicide attempt or episode of self-harm

Male gender

Living alone

Inadequate social support

Life events involving loss (e.g., bereavement) and negative events

Chronic stressors (e.g., environmental or financial)

Chronic medical conditions, including cancer (especially if painful)

Alcohol misuse

Rigid personality styles

Cultural acceptability (in some societies, suicide is more acceptable than in others)

Illness factors

Mental disorder (any mood disorder, psychosis, or substance misuse)

Agitation

Insomnia

Guilt

Hopelessness

Low self-esteem

Hypochondriacal preoccupations

Specific behaviours

Suicide intent or plans expressed

'Accidental' overdose

Leaving notes for those left behind

Altering wills

Hoarding tablets

Severe self-neglect

3.3 Cognitive disturbance in depression

3.3.1 The nature and significance of cognitive impairment in late-life depression

Many patients with late-life major depression have cognitive impairment. It is now recognized that this frequently persists after treatment, probably due to the combined effect of depression and age-related brain changes such as atrophy and vascular disease.

Speed of information processing is impaired in depressive disorder, notably on tasks requiring sustained effort. Poor memory associated with depression usually improves with cueing, whereas in dementia it does not. This is because the earliest (registration) stage of memory is affected, so that the information is not merely difficult to access but non-existent. Functional imaging suggests that the areas of the brain involved in the cognitive disorder of Alzheimer's disease are different from those involved in the cognitive impairment seen in major depression (Dolan *et al.* 1992). However, amnesia and depression can be early symptoms of Alzheimer's disease whilst in chronic depression hypercortisolaemia due to dysregulation of the hypo-pituitary-adrenal axis (HPA) may cause subtle hippocampal damage leading to memory impairment.

Alexopoulos *et al.* (2002) has made note of depression executive dysfunction syndrome (DEDS) in late-life depression. Deficits in higher-order cognition are not usually affected by depression alone, rather there are deficits in executive tasks (planning, initiation, and task persistence) and speed of information processing (Butters *et al.* 2004). Clinically, these patients present with slow inefficient thinking, patchy memory impairment, and are often apathetic. Some regard executive problems as a particular feature of late-onset major depression whilst memory disturbance is possibly more prominent in early-onset cases. This also implies different aetiological pathways: executive dysfunction arising from vascular injury to the FSC and amnesia from neurodegeneration of limbic regions.

Does DEDS or other forms of impaired cognition predict later dementia? Patients with clear deficits in cognition at the outset of their depression do seem to have a higher risk of later dementia. Unfortunately, this seems to be the case even when the impaired cognition recovers as the depression lifts. It is tempting to think that those with DEDS go on to develop vascular dementia whilst those with amnesia may proceed to Alzheimer's disease, but the detailed research to prove this has not yet been performed. Other than patients who present with clear cognitive impairment when depressed, the great majority can be reassured that they are not at risk of dementia.

Epidemiological studies tell us that depression seems to be a risk factor for later cognitive impairment or dementia (Sachs-Ericsson *et al.* 2005). This may be due to mechanisms such as chronically raised cortisol as mentioned, or simply because depression is a common prodromal symptom of dementia. However, these links are associative and cannot be applied to the level of the individual patient.

3.3.2 Differentiating depression from dementia

This important differential diagnosis starts with the history (Table 3.1). Dementia usually begins and proceeds slowly compared with major depression. Typically in dementia, relatives and caregivers are the first to notice memory problems, whereas in depression it is usually the patient who complains of a 'bad' memory. On memory testing, those with dementia may guess answers whilst patients with depression may struggle to summon the effort and simply give up with an 'I don't know'. As discussed, this too reflects the fact that dementia affects higher cortical function, such as higher order memory, whereas depressive disorder affects concentration and information processing, often referred to as 'subcortical'.

Given the importance of making the correct diagnosis, Olin et al. (2002) have proposed criteria for the diagnosis of depression in Alzheimer's disease which include symptoms not emphasized in ICD-10 or DSM-IV, such as reduced positive affect, social isolation, and withdrawal (Box 3.5). Another useful avenue is screening, and the Cornell Scale (see Appendix) was devised to detect depressive disorder in dementia.

Table 3.1 Dementia and depression

Dementia	Depression
Insidious	Rapid onset
Symptoms usually of long duration	Symptoms usually of short duration
Mood and behaviour fluctuate	Mood is consistently depressed
'Near miss' answers typical	'Don't know' answers typical
Patient conceals forgetfulness	Patient highlights forgetfulness
Cognitive impairment relatively stable	Cognitive impairment fluctuates greatly
Higher cortical dysfunction evident	Higher cortical dysfunction absent

Box 3.5 Provisional criteria for depression in Alzheimer's disease

(A) Three (or more) of the following symptoms have been present during the same 2-week period and represent a change from previous functioning: at least one of the symptoms is either (1) depressed mood or (2) decreased positive affect or pleasure.

Note: Do not include symptoms that, in your judgement, are clearly due to a medical condition other than Alzheimer's disease, or are a direct result of non-mood related dementia symptoms (e.g., loss of weight due to difficulties with food intake).

- Clinical significant depressed mood (e.g., depressed, sad, hopeless, discouraged, and tearful)
- Decreased positive affect or pleasure in response to social contacts and usual activities
- Social isolation or withdrawal
- Disruption in appetite
- Disruption in sleep
- Psychomotor changes (e.g., agitation or retardation)
- Irritability
- Fatigue or loss of energy
- Feelings of worthlessness, hopelessness, or excessive or inappropriate guilt
- Recurrent thoughts of death, suicidal ideation, plan, or attempt.

> **Box 3.5** *Contd.*
>
> (B) All criteria are met for dementia of the Alzheimer type.
> (C) The symptoms cause clinically significant distress or disruption in functioning.
> (D) The symptoms do not occur exclusively during the course of a delirium.
> (E) The symptoms are not due to the direct physiological effects of a substance (e.g., a drug of abuse or a medication).
> (F) The symptoms are not better accounted for by other conditions such as a major depressive disorder, bipolar disorder, bereavement, schizophrenia, schizoaffective disorder, psychosis of Alzheimer's disease, anxiety disorders, or substance-related disorder.
>
> After Olin *et al.* (2002).

3.3.3 Depression occurring during established cognitive impairment and dementia

Between 30% and 50% of people with Alzheimer's disease have significant depressive symptoms as do a quarter of those with precursor states such as mild cognitive impairment (Potter and Steffens 2007).

Key references

Alexopoulos GS, Kiosses DN, Klimstra S, Kalayam B, and Bruce ML (2002). Clinical presentation of the "Depression–Executive Dysfunction Syndrome" of late life. *American Journal of Geriatric Psychiatry*, **10**, 98–106.

Baldwin RC (1995). Delusional depression in elderly patients: characteristics and relationship to age at onset. *International Journal of Geriatric Psychiatry*, **10**, 981–5.

Brodaty H, Luscombe G, Parker G, *et al.* (2001). Early and late onset depression in old age: different aetiologies, same phenomenology. *Journal of Affective Disorders*, **66**(2–3), 225–36.

Butters MA, Whyte EM, Nebes RD, *et al.* (2004). The nature and determinants of neuropsychological functioning in late-life depression. *Archives of General Psychiatry*, **61**, 587–95.

Dolan RJ, Bench CJ, Brown RG, Scott LC, Friston KJ, and Frackowiak RSJ (1992). Regional cerebral blood flow abnormalities in depressed patients with cognitive impairment. *Journal of Neurology, Neurosurgery and Psychiatry*, **55**, 768–73.

Koenig HG, George LK, Peterson BL, and Pieper CF (1997). Depression in medically ill hospitalized older adults: prevalence, characteristics, and course of symptoms according to six diagnostic schemes. *American Journal of Psychiatry*, **154**(10), 1376–83.

Olin JT, Schneider LS, Katz IR, *et al.* (2002). Provisional diagnostic criteria for depression of Alzheimer disease. *American Journal of Geriatric Psychiatry*, **10**(2), 125–8.

Pearlson GD, Rabins PV, Kim WS, *et al.* (1989). Structural brain CT changes and cognitive deficits with and without reversible dementia ('pseudodementia'). *Psychological Medicine*, **19**, 573-84.

Potter GG and Steffens DC (2007). Contribution of depression to cognitive impairment and dementia in older adults. *The Neurologist*, **13**, 105–17.

Sachs-Ericsson N, Joiner T, Plant EA, and Blazer DG (2005). The influence of depression on cognitive decline in community-dwelling elderly persons. *American Journal of Geriatric Psychiatry*, **13**, 402–8.

Van Reekum R, Stuss DT, and Ostrander L (2005). Apathy: why care? *The Journal of Neuropsychiatry and Clinical Neurosciences*, **17**, 7–19.

Chapter 4

Aetiology

Key points

- Disability and handicap are closely linked to the aetiology of late-life depressive disorder.
- Always check for underlying physical illness and various prescribed drugs as potential causes of depressive disorder in later life.
- Vascular disease (vascular depression) is increasingly recognized as a cause of late-onset depressive disorder.
- However, in many cases of late-life depression the cause is multifactorial.
- Being a caregiver of someone with dementia is associated with a high risk of depression.

Often there are multiple causes and pathways to depressive disorder in later life. To aid thinking, aetiology can be subdivided into three 'p's': predisposing risk factors, precipitating factors, and perpetuating features (Table 4.1).

4.1 Predisposing factors

4.1.1 Genetic susceptibility

There is less genetic susceptibility to depression in later life than in younger life. An exception is depressive episode occurring as part of bipolar affective disorder, which often recurs in later life and has a strong genetic basis. In contrast to its role in dementia, no definite role has been established for the ε4 allele of the apolipoprotein E gene in the origin of late-life depression.

4.1.2 Gender and civil status

At all ages, depression is more frequent in women, especially in widows and divorcees.

Table 4.1 Factors involved in the causation of late-life depression

Predisposing	Precipitating	Perpetuating	Protective
Genes (minimal)	Adverse life events (usually of loss)	Poor health	Adaptive coping style
Gender and civil status	Chronic stress and difficulties	Social adversity	Resilience
Past psychiatric history	Medication	Handicap	Affiliation (e.g., religious group)
Physical ill-health, impairment, and handicap		Poor social support	High level of perceived support
Sensory impairment		Relationship and family difficulties	Positive life events
Personality (avoidant, dependent, obsessional)			
Psychosocial (poverty, crime, and loneliness)			
Degree of acculturation			
Caregiving			

4.1.3 **Past psychiatric history**

A past history of depressive disorder or dysthymic disorder is an undoubted risk factor for late-life depression (Cole and Dendukuri 2003). Alcohol dependency and schizophrenia are associated with depression.

4.1.4 **Physical ill-health, impairment, and handicap**

The interaction between ill health and depressive disorders is complex and bidirectional; chronic ill health can predispose to depression as well as worsen its prognosis, and the presence of a depressive disorder can also worsen the outcome of physical illness. A vicious cycle may establish itself in which physical impairment provokes depression, which may in turn add to the disability of the original impairing condition (Prince et al. 1998).

Other factors associated with ageing such as hearing and visual loss predispose to depressive disorder (Rovner et al. 2007). In addition, frequent primary care attendance and a high level of home support are possible markers for depressive disorder (Katona and Shankar 2004).

Ischaemic heart disease, several neurological disorders (such as Parkinson's disease and Alzheimer's disease), cerebrovascular disease (such as vascular dementia and stroke), hip fracture, and chronic obstructive pulmonary disease have all been associated with a high level of depression in older adults (Blazer 2003; Alexopoulos 2005). Pain syndromes, with various causes, are also closely linked to depression. Again, these associations are bidirectional: depression worsens pain and pain leads to depression. A range of disorders, some not obvious at presentation, can predispose to depressive disorder (see Table 4.2). Co-morbidity is considered in more detail in Chapter 5.

Table 4.2 Medical conditions and central-acting drugs that may cause organic depressive disorder	
Medical conditions	Central-acting drugs
Endocrine/metabolic	**Antihypertensive drugs**
Diabetes	β-Blockers (especially non-selective)
Hypo-/hyperthyroidism	Methyldopa
Cushing's disease	Reserpine
Hypercalcaemia	Clonidine
Sub-nutrition	Nifedipine, calcium channel agents
Pernicious anaemia	Digoxin
Organic brain disease	**Steroids**
Cerebrovascular disease/stroke	**Analgesic drugs**
CNS tumours	Opioids
Parkinson's disease	Indometacin
Alzheimer's disease/vascular dementia	**Antiparkinson**
Multiple sclerosis	Levodopa
Systemic lupus erythematosus	Amantadine
Occult carcinoma	Tetrabenazine
Pancreas	**Psychiatric drugs**
Lung	Neuroleptics
Chronic infections	Benzodiazepines
Neurosyphilis	**Miscellaneous**
Brucellosis	Sulfonamides
Neurocysticercosis	Alcohol
Myalgic encephalomyelitis	Interferon
AIDS	

There are several mechanisms whereby medical conditions may lead to depression. For the neurological disorders such as the dementias, stroke, and Parkinson's disease, alteration in the brain serotonergic systems may be important. However, the wide range of disabling medical conditions which seem to increase vulnerability to depression suggests that the meaning of the illness for the sufferer is as important as the precise organ system involved. Prince *et al.* (1998) have shown that the concept of handicap—the disadvantage in society resulting from impairment and disability—is an important risk factor for depression in older people. This concept not only helps understand depression but also emphasizes that handicap is as much a societal issue as a medical one. Two older people may be similarly impaired by medical illnesses but if one has limited practical support and poor access to transport, then he/she is the more handicapped. The implications for treating depression are obvious.

4.1.5 **Personality and developmental factors**

Structured personality assessment suggests that personality dysfunction, especially of the 'avoidant' and 'dependent' types, is associated with late-life depression (Blazer and Hybels 2005). Murphy (1982) found that a lack of a capacity for intimacy life-long, which is probably a personality trait, was a risk factor for depression in later life. Character and personality traits also interact with life events to modify the risk of depression. Positive coping styles, self-efficacy, and a high level of mastery over the environment are the traits that protect the individual from depression (Blazer and Hybels 2005) (Table 4.1).

In one study, 'Cluster C' personality traits (meaning avoidant, dependent, perfectionist, and/or self-defeating in nature) influenced the outcome of depressive disorder in patients aged 60 and above. Compared to patients with non-'Cluster C' personality, those with the trait were as likely to respond to treatment but did so more slowly and experienced greater functional impairment (Morse and Robins 2005). This exemplifies the idea of multiple factors, both organic and non-organic, influencing depression and, in this case, pointing towards specific groups of patients who might benefit from a psychological intervention in addition to an antidepressant. Given the limited availability of psychological therapies this could be important.

The increased awareness of childhood abuse, including sexual abuse, as a risk factor for depression should not be overlooked just because the patient is older. Strategies that may have enabled coping with adversity earlier in life may break down under ill-health, loss, or other threatening life events, resurrecting memories of abuse.

4.1.6 **Psychosocial factors**

Poverty, poor social support, and social isolation are risk factors for depression in later life. A vicious cycle can be engendered as low socio-economic status and low access to appropriate treatments tend to go together (Arean and Reynolds 2005). Being a victim of crime is also linked to socio-economic status, making it too a risk factor (Arean and Reynolds 2005). The fear of becoming a victim of crime may be almost as disabling as becoming one since fear reinforces lifestyles which promote depression, such as isolation and avoidance of outside activity.

4.1.7 Ethnic and cultural factors

Acculturation refers to how individuals respond to a dominant culture. This affects the detection of depression, the uptake of mental health services, and the acceptability of treatment. Among older adults, lower levels of acculturation typically lead to a lower likelihood of detecting depression and lower rates of usage of antidepressants. Among ethnic minorities, barriers to the acceptance of mental health care include stigma, concerns about financial reimbursement (in some health systems), limited geographical access to specialist mental health services, distrust of mental health providers, and culturally inappropriate services (Unützer et al. 1999).

4.1.8 Caregiving

Given the increase in dementia and long-term medical conditions in the population, this deserves emphasis as a risk factor for depression. Ballard et al. (1996) reported a quarter of caregivers of those with dementia were depressed and many had persistent symptoms. Factors associated with depression in caregivers include depression in the designated patient and problem behaviours. Financial strain adds to the risk (Blazer and Hybels 2005).

4.2 Precipitating factors

4.2.1 Life events

Table 4.3 lists the more common life events and stressors associated with late-life depressive disorder. In a population of 119 people suffering from depressive disorder, Murphy (1982) found that 48% had experienced at least one severe life event in the preceding year compared to 23% of a control group. These were threatening and often involved loss, including bereavement due to the loss of someone close or even a loved pet, life threatening illness to oneself or someone close; major financial problems; and having to give up one's home suddenly, usually after a serious illness. In addition, major social difficulties (as distinct from sudden events) lasting for 2 years or more were also significantly associated with depression.

If adversity alone was sufficient to 'explain' depression then eventually all old people would fall victim to it. Yet a quarter of Murphy's

Table 4.3 Common causes of depression: life events and chronic stress

Life events	Chronic stress
Bereavement	Declining health and mobility; dependence
Separation	
Acute physical illness	Sensory loss, cognitive decline
Medical illness or threat to life of someone close	Housing problems
	Major problems affecting family member
Sudden homelessness or having to move into a care home	
	Marital difficulties
Major financial crisis	Socio-economic decline
Negative interactions with family member or friend	Problems at work; retirement
Loss of 'significant other' (including a pet)	Caring for a chronically ill and dependent family member

control group had suffered a major adverse life event and did not develop depression. Not all adverse events are followed by depression; not all depressions are preceded by adverse life events. An uncritical acceptance that a particular life event 'caused' depression can lead to overlooking a hidden medical problem which may be the real cause.

Bereavement is a common trigger for depressive disorder in later life. The symptoms of grief and depression often overlap. In brief, in the first month low mood, anorexia, insomnia, crying bouts, fatigue, loss of interest, and guilt are common. The latter is typically a rumination about what might have been done to save the person. Suicidal thinking is rare at this stage. After 12 months, somatic symptoms have usually improved although low mood and poor sleep may persist. The persistence of earlier symptoms is one sign that a bereavement is now complicated by depressive disorder. Other symptoms associated with depression complicating grief include suicidal thoughts or wishing oneself dead, pervasive guilt (not merely remorse over what more might have been done to prevent death), persistent feelings of worthlessness or hopelessness, 'mummification' (maintaining grief by keeping everything the same), and psychomotor retardation.

Criterion E of Box 2.1 (DSM) has been interpreted to mean that when symptoms of major depression arise within 2 months of a bereavement and do not persist beyond these 2 months, a diagnosis of major depression should not be made, unless the symptoms are associated with marked impairment or include morbid preoccupation such as the one described earlier. This may change in the next revision of DSM as it becomes clearer that bereavement-related depression resembles depression unrelated to bereavement and that the treatment response appears similar. However, it is important not to pathologize normal human reactions so that a considerable degree of clinical judgement will be required. The issue is of obvious importance to older adults who experience high levels of bereavement.

4.2.2 Medication

Many medications (Table 4.2) are associated with depression, although it is difficult to prove a causal relationship. In a study from Holland, Dhondt et al. (2002) examined a large epidemiological database and found that non-selective β-blockers, calcium antagonists, systemic steroids, and benzodiazepines were all aetiologically relevant to late-life depression. Self-medication with alcohol may lead to depression or aggravate it.

4.3 Protective factors

Relatively little is known about factors that protect against late-life depression (Table 4.1). If lack of a confidant leads to depression (Murphy 1982), does the availability of close relationships offer protection from depression? What seems to matter is not merely the availability of such relationships but whether they are perceived as close and supportive (Blazer and Hybels 2005).

Adaptive coping styles and psychological resilience are further individual factors which may lessen the chances of depression after adversity or stress (Arean and Reynolds 2005). Resilience means the ability to make sense of events, accept one's existence, and carry on with life.

Affiliation and belonging are also important. Religious observance has been shown to protect against depression in older adults in both Western and Eastern cultures (Blazer 2003). Positive events, such as a new grandchild, may protect against depression.

4.4 Neurobiological factors in late-life depression

Although there are multiple pathways to depression, the final changes must occur in the brain. This section covers what is known about the brain in late-life depression.

The biological theory of depression dates back to the 1960 with amine hypothesis which proposed that brain deficiency of noradrenaline and serotonin (5-HT) caused depression. Nowadays, the emphasis is on neurotransmitter systems rather than single chemicals. These include dopamine pathways, corticotropin-releasing factor (CRF), thyrotropin-releasing hormone, and growth hormone releasing factor, along with their associated neurohormonal systems, such as the hypothalamic-pituitary-adrenal (HPA) axis. The role of immune and inflammatory responses is also increasingly recognized since complex interactions occur between the HPA axis and the immune and inflammatory systems.

4.4.1 **Biogenic amines**

Noradrenaline is associated with attention, memory, concentration, and states of arousal; serotonin with impulse control, sex drive, appetite, and mood; whilst dopamine is concerned with motivation, hedonia, exploratory behaviour, and reward-mediated behaviour from activities such as food, sex, and social interaction. It seems reasonable to postulate that amine deficiency might increasingly occur with age. In fact this is controversial. More sophisticated understanding of depression has shifted to knowledge of receptor function. For example, autoreceptor binding was dysfunctional in one study of late-life depression and associated with failure to respond to antidepressant medication (Meltzer et al. 2004).

4.4.2 **Neuroendocrine changes**

At all ages, depression is associated with hyperactivity and dysregulation of the HPA axis. Ageing is associated with increasing cortisol levels and cortisol nonsuppression. As mentioned earlier, hippocampal atrophy has been linked to chronic depression via cortisol stress. Corticotropin-releasing hormone (CRH) is secreted by the hypothalamus and it has been shown that CRH mRNA levels in the paraventricular nucleus of elderly depressed patients are higher than the levels in Alzheimer's disease patients (also elevated), and very much higher than normal controls (Raadsheer et al. 1995). This has led to speculation that hyperactivation of paraventricular CRH neurons may contribute to the aetiology of late-life depression.

Early life trauma may lead to long-term hypersensitivity of the HPA and CRF systems, which is the basis of the 'stress-diathesis' model of depression. Genetic disposition coupled with early stress in critical phases of development may lead an individual to be more vulnerable to developing depression and anxiety upon further exposure to stress. In a study of over 800 singletons born in the 1920s who were interviewed at an average age of 68, Thompson et al. (2001) found that the odds ratio for depression among men, but not women, rose incrementally with decreasing birth weight. This could be mediated by faulty programming of the HPA axis very early in life.

4.4.3 **Immune and inflammatory changes**

Excessive or prolonged exposure to glucocorticoids can compromise the immune system and mechanisms of inflammation. In late-life depression, there is evidence of increase in pro-inflammatory markers but it is not known which came first, the inflammatory changes or the depression (Teper and O'Brien 2007).

4.4.4 The vascular depression hypothesis

For many years, clinicians have suspected that cerebrovascular disease may be relevant to late-life depression. The vascular depression hypothesis proposes that vascular brain disease may predispose to, precipitate, or perpetuate late-life depression (Alexopoulos 2005). Features of vascular depression include less depressive ideation, more psychomotor retardation, poorer insight, executive dysfunction, greater disability, and an onset usually after aged 60. In addition, magnetic resonance imaging (MRI) has shown that patients with late-life depression have a higher rate of hyperintensities in the deep white matter and basal ganglia compared to control subjects, with the greatest effects seen in late-onset cases. These data have been supplemented by large epidemiological studies which confirm that the severity and location (especially in the basal ganglia) of white matter lesions (WML) are likely to be of causal relevance in late-life depression, as reviewed by Baldwin, 2005.

Although there are several causes of WML, a reasonable assumption is that in depressed patients they reflect cerebral ischaemia. However, a clear cut association between the symptoms of vascular depression and common cerebrovascular risk factors (such as hypertension, smoking, hyperlipidaemia, and diabetes) has not been shown nor is there a consistent relationship between cerebrovascular risk factors and depression severity, symptomatology, or brain volume measures (Baldwin 2005). This does not rule out ischaemia since chronic hypoperfusion (rather than infarction) may be the causal problem. Brain hypoperfusion is not readily detected by 'bedside' measures of cerebrovascular function other than perhaps postural hypotension, so more sophisticated research will be needed.

The presence of WML - especially when numerous, severe in extent, or strategically located (as in the basal ganglia - is also of relevance to a poorer outcome for depression in later life (Baldwin 2005). If a significant proportion of late-life depression has a vascular basis, then vasoprotective treatment might possibly help depression. One study has shown that in patients with late-life depression nimodipine, a drug with vasoprotective properties, when combined with antidepressant medication, led to a reduced time to remission and a longer time before recurrence compared with a placebo augmentation (Tarangano et al. 2005). This needs to be replicated before such drugs can be recommended.

The vascular depression hypothesis has its critics. Nevertheless, there is strong evidence (to be discussed in Chapter 5) that vascular disease and depression are linked in a bidirectional manner, each increasing the risk of the other. The vascular depression hypothesis may ultimately prove too restrictive from a conceptual point of view, but clinically it serves as a reminder that patient management should encompass both psychiatric symptoms and medical co-morbidity such as vascular disease.

4.4.5 Neurodegeneration

Early studies with computerized tomography (CT) showed that brain atrophy occurs in patients with late-life depression. Atrophy and ischaemia probably represent alternate pathways to depression (Baldwin 2005).

4.4.6 Functional imaging and EEG

The electroencephalogram (EEG) is not a useful investigation in depression unless to help rule out organic brain disease such as a delirium or dementia. The P300 paradigm uses evoked responses to assess physiological correlates of psychomotor slowing via the EEG. It is an event-related potential recorded via the EEG in the form of a positive deflection in voltage at a latency of ~300ms in the EEG. It may serve as a proxy for superior limbic function, and longer latencies have been found in late-life depression with executive dysfunction. This interesting technology has not yet found an application in clinical practice.

Abnormalities in regional cerebral blood flow using positron emission tomography (PET) in middle-aged and elderly depressed subjects have been reported (Bench et al. 1992). Regions particularly affected are the left anterior cingulate gyrus and left dorsolateral prefrontal cortex. As mentioned in the previous chapter, in patients with both depression and cognitive impairment, reduced flow to the left anterior medial prefrontal gyrus and increased flow to the cerebellar vermis occur. Such distinct differences in patterns of blood perfusion in depressed patients with and without cognitive impairment help in the understanding of the cerebral basis of altered cognition in depression.

Single photon emission computerized tomography (SPECT) uses a radioactive tracer, such as ^{99}Tc-hexamethylpropylene amine oxime. There are few studies of older depressed patients but there is some evidence for a reduction in cerebral perfusion mainly involving the frontal cortex (Bench et al. 1992).

It is now recognized that distributed neuronal networks and not just single pathways or neurochemicals are important in depression. Tekin and Cummings (2002) have suggested that superior limbic structures may regulate attention and cognitive aspects of depression (apathy, psychomotor disturbance, impaired attention, and dysexecutive symptoms); a ventral compartment formed of limbic, paralimbic, and subcortical structures may mediate vegetative and somatic aspects (sleep, appetite, endocrine disturbance); and the rostral cingulate area may regulate interactions between these two.

4.4.7 **Post-mortem findings**

The deep white matter hyperintensities of late-life depression visualized on MRI have correlates in brain post-mortem tissue where they are revealed to be ischaemic in origin (summarized by Baldwin 2005; Teper and O'Brien 2007). Ischaemic WML tended to be found mainly in the dorsolateral prefrontal cortex which fits with the PET data above.

Finally, since there are multiple pathways to depression in later life, Figure 4.1 illustrates how some of these pathways may interact to cause depression. To support the multiple pathway view of late-life depression, van den Berg *et al.* (2001) studied 132 older depressed patients and found three distinct pathways: an early-onset group associated with a family history and neuroticism, a late-onset group associated with severe life stresses, and a late-onset group associated with vascular risk factors.

Figure 4.1 Pathways to depression

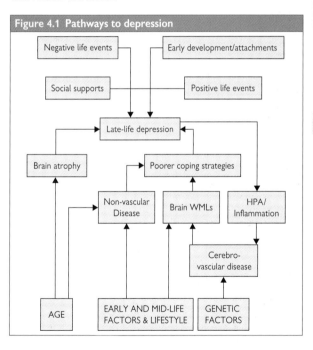

Key references

Alexopoulos GS (2005). Depression in the elderly. *The Lancet*, **365**(9475), 1961–70.

Arean PA and Reynolds CF (2005). The impact of psychosocial factors on late-life depression. *Biological Psychiatry*, **58**, 277–82.

Baldwin RC (2005). Is vascular depression a distinct sub-type of depressive disorder? A review of causal evidence. *International Journal of Geriatric Psychiatry*, **20**, 1–11.

Ballard CG, Eastwood C, Gahir M, and Wilcock G (1996). A follow-up study of depression in the carers of dementia sufferers. *British Medical Journal*, **312**, 947.

Bench CJ, Friston KJ, Brown RG, Scott LC, Frackowiak RSJ, Dolan RJ (1992). The anatomy of depression - focal abnormalities of cerebral blood flow in major depression. *Psychological Medicine*, **22**, 607–15.

Blazer DG (2003). Depression in late life: review and commentary. *Journal of Gerontology: Medical Sciences*, **58A**, 249–65.

Blazer DG II and Hybels CF (2005). Origin of depression in later life. *Psychological Medicine*, 35, 1241–52.

Cole MG and Dendukuri N (2003). Risk factors for elderly community subjects: a systematic review and meta-analysis. *American Journal of Psychiatry*, **160**, 1147–56.

Dhondt TDF, Beekman ATF, Deeg DJH, and van Tilburg W (2002). Iatrogenic depression in the elderly: results from a community-based study in the Netherlands. *Social Psychiatry and Psychiatric Epidemiology*, **37**, 393–8.

Katona CLE and Shankar KK (2004). Depression in old age. *Reviews in Clinical Gerontology*, **14**, 283–306.

Meltzer CC, Price JC, Mathis CA, *et al.* (2004). Serotonin 1A receptor binding and treatment response in late-life depression. *Neuropsychopharmacology*, **29**(12), 2258–65.

Morse JQ and Robins CJ (2005). Personality-life event congruence effects in late-life depression. *Journal of Affective Disorders*, **84**(1), 25–31.

Murphy E (1982). Social origins of depression in old age. *British Journal of Psychiatry*, **141**, 135–42.

Prince MJ, Harwood RH, Thomas A, and Mann AH (1998). A prospective population-based cohort study of the effects of disablement and social milieu on the onset and maintenance of late-life depression. The Gospel Oak Project VII. *Psychological Medicine*, **28**, 337–50.

Raadsheer FC, Joop J, Van Heerikhuize JJ, and Lucassen PJ (1995). Corticotropin-releasing hormone mRNA levels in the paraventricular nucleus of patients with Alzheimer's disease and depression. *Archives of General Psychiatry*, **152**, 1372–6.

Rovner BW, Casten RJ, and Hegel MT (2007). Preventing depression in age-related macular degeneration. *Archives of General Psychiatry*, **64**(8), 886–92.

Tarangano FE, Bagnatti P, and Allegri RF (2005). A double-blind, randomized clinical trial to assess the augmentation with nimodipine of antidepressant therapy in the treatment of vascular depression. *International Psychogeriatrics*, **17**, 487–98.

Tekin S and Cummings JL (2002). Frontal-subcortical neuronal circuits and clinical neuropsychiatry: an update. *Journal of Psychosomatic Research*, **53**, 647–54.

Teper E and O'Brien JT (2007). Vascular factors and depression. *International Journal of Geriatric Psychiatry*, **23**, 993–1000.

Thompson C, Syddall H, Rodin I, Osmond C, and Barker DJP (2001). Birth weight and the risk of depressive disorder in late life. *The British Journal of Psychiatry*, **179**, 450–5.

Unützer J, Katon W, Sullivan M, and Miranda J (1999). Treating depressed older adults in primary care: narrowing the gap between efficacy and effectiveness. *The Millbank Quarterly*, **77**, 225–56.

Van den Berg MD, Oldehinkel AJ, Bouhuys AL, Brilman EI, Beekman ATF, and Ormel J (2001). Depression in later life: three etiologically different subgroups. *Journal of Affective Disorders*, **65**, 19–26.

Chapter 5

Co-morbidity and depression in late life

> **Key points**
> - A number of physical illnesses common in older people are associated with high levels of depressive disorder.
> - There is considerable evidence that depression predisposes to vascular disease.
> - The relationship between depression and vascular disease is two-way.

Co-morbidity, whether from medical illness or cognitive impairment, is at the heart of old age psychiatry. This chapter considers how these areas interlink in specific conditions that are common in older people: stroke, cardiac disease, diabetes mellitus, Parkinson's disease, chronic obstructive pulmonary disease (COPD), cancer, and pain. Management will be covered in Chapter 6.

5.1 Cognitive impairment

As discussed earlier, depression is highly prevalent in dementia and chronic depression is a risk factor for dementia, a risk that is possibly increased by the presence of the Apolipoprotein E (APOE) ε4 allele. Depression can also be a prodromal symptom of dementia. A cut-off of around 10 years has been suggested, within which depression may be a prodromal symptom of dementia but beyond which it is a risk factor for dementia.

5.2 Stroke and mood disorder

5.2.1 Depression

Depression develops in around 20% of patients within the first year after a stroke, with peak prevalence at 3–6 months, tailing off after 2 or 3 years (Paranthaman and Baldwin 2006). Post-stroke depression has been shown to be a predictor of impaired quality of life and a risk factor for cognitive decline and poorer functional recovery (Evans *et al.*

2005). Making a diagnosis of depression after a stroke can be difficult, especially in patients with aphasia. The 14-item observer-rated Stroke Aphasic Depression Questionnaire Hospital Version (SADQ-H) is one option (Bennett and Lincoln 2006).

Predisposing factors for post-stroke depression include older age, a history of depressive disorder, the size of infarct, female sex, residual disability, and language impairment. Whether baseline depressive symptoms predict later cerebrovascular events is controversial and it may depend on how rigorously researchers have controlled the effects of pre-existent vascular risk factors such as smoking. How depression might predispose to stroke is not fully understood but depression is known to affect autonomic function and platelet activation.

Difficulty in adjusting to major disability may be sufficient to trigger depression. However, the very high rate of depression and the fact that the relationship between objective severity of stroke and depression is not a consistent one has led to a localization hypothesis. Specifically, it has been suggested that lesions closer to the anterior pole of the left hemisphere are a risk factor for depression, possibly via the disruption of routes connecting the brainstem with the cortex, although not all agree with the localization hypothesis (Evans *et al.* 2005).

5.2.2 Post-stroke emotionalism

Emotional changes following stroke have been variously described as 'emotionalism', 'pathological affect', 'lability of mood', and emotional 'incontinence'. In emotionalism, crying (or rarely laughing) comes with little or no warning and is hard to control, so that the subject cries or laughs in social situations where she or he would not previously have done. It affects 20%–25% of survivors in the first 6 months after stroke (Paranthaman and Baldwin 2006). Although it declines in frequency and severity over the first year, at 12 months about 10%–15% of survivors remain affected, with some having persistent severe problems. Depressed mood and emotionalism can occur together, but most people with emotionalism are not depressed. It can occur following a single cortical stroke or bilateral subcortical strokes. There may be a link to serotonergic mechanisms as lesions have been noted more commonly in the raphae nuclei, which is an area rich in serotonergic neurons (Paranthaman and Baldwin 2006).

5.3 Coronary heart disease

Depressive symptoms occur in about 15%–20% soon after a coronary event (Evans *et al.* 2005). At 2 months of 804 patients with stable coronary heart disease (CHD), 7.1% met criteria for major depression and 5.3% for generalized anxiety disorder (Frasure-Smith and Lespérance 2008). These rates are much higher compared to the general population.

An epidemiological study of older adults from Holland showed that cardiac patients with minor (sub-threshold) depression had a relative risk of subsequent cardiac mortality of 1.6 rising to 3.0 for those with major depression, after adjustment for confounding factors (Penninx et al. 2001). Negative effects on cardiac outcome are seen whether or not subjects are healthy at baseline and can last for many years but the maximum impact is generally within the first year after an acute myocardial infarct.

The evidence for depression as an independent risk factor for vascular events has been sufficiently robust for the American Heart Association to recommend screening for depression in cardiac patients. A caution though is that adjustment for baseline factors, especially left ventricular function, substantially attenuates the association of depression and CHD so that 'reverse causality' (those with more severe baseline CHD being more likely to report depression) cannot be ruled out.

5.3.1 Possible mechanisms

Biological explanations include autonomic imbalance, known to be associated with major depression, leading to sympathetic overactivity and/or parasympathetic under-activity, with decreased heart rate variability, down-regulated beta-adrenergic receptors, and decreased baroreflex sensitivity, making the diseased heart more susceptible to arrhythmias. Autonomic imbalance is an independent risk factor for early cardiovascular mortality (Carney et al. 2007). Platelets may be more activated in depressed patients with heart disease than in depressed patients without heart disease. The vascular endothelium produces local vasoactive agents, including nitric oxide (a vasodilator) and the peptide endothelin (a vasoconstrictor). Endothelial dysfunction is thought to precede and predict atheroma and there is evidence of impairment in adults with depressive disorder. Lifestyle factors in depression include a reduced likelihood of taking medication such as antihypertensives and antidepressants, inactivity, lack of exercise, smoking, and excessive alcohol intake. These may mediate the relationship between depression and vascular disease (Figure 5.1). Finally, those with vascular disease may subtly recognize that something is wrong before it becomes clinically apparent, thereby triggering depression.

5.3.2 Important variables

That depression is bad for arteries is shown by the Pittsburgh Healthy Heart Project (Stewart et al. 2007) which indicated that among 324 adults aged 50–70 years, higher depressive symptoms at baseline were associated with greater 3-year change in carotid intima-media thickness (a measure of atheroma) after adjusting for confounding factors.

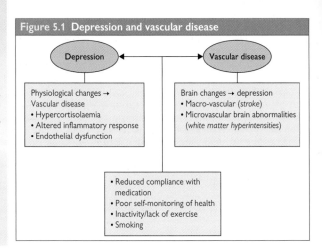

Figure 5.1 Depression and vascular disease

Depression ↔ Vascular disease

Physiological changes → Vascular disease
• Hypercortisolaemia
• Altered inflammatory response
• Endothelial dysfunction

Brain changes → depression
• Macro-vascular (stroke)
• Microvascular brain abnormalities (white matter hyperintensities)

• Reduced compliance with medication
• Poor self-monitoring of health
• Inactivity/lack of exercise
• Smoking

5.4 Diabetes

The frequency of type 2 diabetes increases with age. In a cohort of patients aged 70–79 years followed for about 6 years, those with diabetes had an increased level of depression which attenuated after adjustment for diabetes-related co-morbidities, although this still represented a significantly increased risk compared to controls. In this study, HbA1c was a predictor of recurrent depression (Maraldi et al. 2007).

There is some evidence of a link between depression and the occurrence of diabetic complications and poorer glycaemic control. Painful neuropathy may be another trigger for depression. Diabetes can cause small vessel pathology in the brain that leads to subcortical encephalopathy, not unlike that seen in vascular depression. This may lead to both cognitive impairment and depressed mood.

5.5 Parkinson's disease

Parkinson's disease causes slowness of movement, rigidity, resting tremor, shuffling gait, and postural instability. Depression in patients with Parkinson's disease is associated with increased physical disability, impaired quality of life, and decreased social interaction.

Slowness of thought ('bradyphrenia') parallels the physical slowness, the risk of dementia is increased and significant depressive symptoms occur in about 40% of patients over the course of the illness (Allain et al. 2000). The depression in these patients differs from primary major depression in that marked negative ideation (self-blame, guilt, feeling a failure, and suicidal thoughts) are less frequent. Also, depressive symptoms precede those of motor dysfunction in 12%–37% of patients (Allain *et al*. 2000) and they contribute to cognitive impairment.

Various causes (biological, psychological, social) combine to produce depression in Parkinson's disease. Functional neuroimaging has identified greater reduction in both serotonin and dopamine pathways in depressed versus non-depressed Parkinson's patients. Other factors include social isolation, cognitive impairment, severity of Parkinson's disease, and duration of illness, although there is an inconsistent relationship between the later two and depression.

5.6 **Chronic obstructive pulmonary disease**

The prevalence of depression in COPD is about 40% and, untreated, it is associated with increased physical disability, impaired quality of life, increased health care use, and a higher risk of death.

How depression is linked to COPD is unclear. Possible mechanisms include factors related to COPD (level of physical disability and fluctuating mood because of dyspnoea), smoking (which increases the risk of vascular brain disease and perhaps 'vascular depression'), and behavioural factors (lack of exercise, limited activity, and associated social isolation). Social factors are important, including disruption to social networks caused by repeated hospital admissions (moderate-to-severe COPD leads to 3–4 admissions per year) or becoming housebound either through worsening disability or the need for continuous oxygen treatment.

5.7 **Cancer and pain**

Both cancer and pain are common in older patients and depression is a frequent co-morbid condition. Depression can precede a diagnosis of cancer, notably lung and pancreatic cancer, and high rates of depression are seen in breast cancer and head and neck tumours (Evans *et al*. 2005).

Simply being given a diagnosis of cancer plus the arduous, distressing nature of treatment along with pain leads to more contact with mental health services (Evans *et al*. 2005). Besides this, anticancer treatment may trigger depression, and cancer may lead to an increase in pro-inflammatory cytokines which have been linked to depression in later life.

Whether depression increases the risk of cancer is controversial but this has been reported in epidemiological research involving older people (Evans *et al.* 2005). One explanation is that depression may work as an immunosuppressant.

In summary, physical illness is commonly associated with depression. There are particular links between depression and both subcortical brain disease and vascular disorder. With regard to the latter, Mast *et al.* (2008) found that it was the cumulative burden of vascular risk and disease rather than individual conditions which significantly predicted future depressive symptoms.

Key references

Allain H, Schuck S, and Maudit N (2000). Depression in Parkinson's disease. *British Medical Journal*, **320**, 1287–8.

Bennett HE and Lincoln NB (2006). Potential screening measures for depression and anxiety after stroke. *International Journal of Therapy and Rehabilitation*, **13**, 401–6.

Carney RM, Freedland KE, Stein PK, *et al.* (2007). Heart rate variability and markers of inflammation and coagulation in depressed patients with coronary heart disease. *British Medical Journal*, **62**, 463–7.

Evans DL, Charney DS, Lewis L, *et al.* (2005). Mood disorders in the medically ill: scientific review and recommendations. *Biological Psychiatry*, **58**, 175–89.

Frasure-Smith N and Lespérance F (2008). Depression and anxiety as predictors of 2-year cardiac events in patients with stable coronary artery disease. *Archives of General Psychiatry*, **65**, 62–71.

Maraldi C, Volpato S, Penninx BW, *et al.* (2007). Diabetes mellitus, glycemic control, and incident depressive symptoms among 70- to 79-year-old persons: the health, aging, and body composition study. *Archives of Internal Medicine*, **167**, 1137–44.

Mast BT, Miles T, Penninx BW, *et al.* (2008). Vascular disease and future risk of depressive symptomatology in older adults: findings from the health, aging, and body composition study. *Biological Psychiatry*; **64**, 320–6.

Paranthaman R and Baldwin RC (2006). Treatments of psychiatric syndromes due to cerebrovascular disease. *International Review of Psychiatry*, **18**(5), 453–70.

Penninx BWJH, Beekman ATF, Honig A, *et al.* (2001). Depression and cardiac mortality results from a community-based longitudinal study. *Archives of General Psychiatry*, **58**, 221–7.

Stewart JS, Janicki DL, Muldoon MF, Sutton-Tyrrell K, and Kamarck TW (2007). Negative emotions and 3-year progression of subclinical atherosclerosis. *Archives of General Psychiatry*, **64**, 225–33.

Chapter 6

Assessment and management

Key points

- Antidepressant drugs are effective in older patients with depressive episode, with no important differences in individual drug efficacy.
- Antidepressants are effective in depressed patients with a range of physical co-morbid conditions, although tolerability varies.
- Age should not be a barrier to receiving a psychological therapy.
- For chronic depression, combining antidepressant medication with a psychological intervention is associated with the best chance of recovery.
- CBT requires only modest modification for older people.
- Supportive psychotherapy is not 'doing nothing'.

6.1 Goals of treatment

Antidepressants, psychological interventions, and electroconvulsive therapy (ECT) all work in older patients just as they do in younger ones. The goals of treatment are to achieve symptomatic remission and to help the patient achieve optimum function, both physically and socially (Baldwin et al. 2002) (Table 6.1). Remission means that the patient is back to normal, not just improved. Residual symptoms predispose to relapse and chronicity. For patients with more intractable symptoms or whose care is complex, attaining optimum function will require input from health professionals such as occupational therapy, physiotherapy, specialist nursing (such as Community Psychiatric Nurses), and social work. This may require referral to specialist psychiatric services. Keeping the patient well after recovery is a further goal and discussed in Chapter 9.

Table 6.1 Goals of treatment of depression	
Goal	**Ways to achieve**
Risk reduction - of suicide or harm from self-neglect	• A risk assessment and monitoring of risk • Prompt referral of urgent cases to a specialist
Remission of all depressive symptoms	• Providing appropriate treatment (usually an antidepressant and/or a psychological treatment) • Giving the patient and his/her supporters timely education about depression and its treatment
To help the patient achieve optimal function	• Enable practical support • Ensure access to appropriate agencies to help
To treat the whole person, including somatic problems	• Treat co-existing physical health problems • Reduce wherever possible the effects of handicap caused by factors such as chronic disease, sensory impairment, and poor mobility • Observe good prescribing practice for older people (6.3.1)
To prevent relapse and recurrence	• Educate the patient about staying on medication once feeling better • Continuation treatment (staying on treatment after recovery) • Maintenance treatment (preventative treatment)

In the United Kingdom, the 'stepped care' model is used (NICE 2004), meaning that treatment is delivered through a series of steps ranging from low-intensity/non-specialist care to high-intensity/specialist input depending on the severity and complexity of the case (see also Chapter 7). Working in collaboration with the patient and offering treatment choice wherever possible underpin effective management.

6.2 Assessing the patient

6.2.1 General assessment

Assessment starts with the history of symptoms and the mental state examination. It is important to screen for cognitive impairment. This can be undertaken by using the Mini-Mental State Examination (MMSE) (Folstein *et al.* 1975) or the briefer 6-item Orientation Memory-Concentration (OMC) (Brooke and Bullock 1999) (see also Chapter 7). A physical examination focused on clues from the history should be carried out; for example, neurological examination in patients complaining of cognitive impairment. Laboratory investigation (Table 6.2) should include haemoglobin and red blood cell counts, which may point to B_{12} deficiency or alcohol misuse. B_{12} and folate estimation should be undertaken in a first episode. Red cell folate gives more information regarding long-term folate stores. Older people decompensate quite quickly as they have limited physiological reserve, the resulting severe depression leads to undernutrition or dehydration. These changes occur much more rapidly than in younger patients. Elevated levels of calcium are occasionally associated with depression, as in primary hyperparathyroidism or metastatic cancer, both of which can cause depressed mood even before the underlying diagnosis is made. Hypothyroidism may be overlooked in the elderly and 'apathetic hyperthyroidism' can be mistaken for depression. In theory, neurosyphilis can cause depression. This is exceedingly rare nowadays, although the incidence of syphilis is once again on the increase in some countries. There should be an adequate clinical reason for conducting neurosyphilis testing in a patient presenting with depression, for example, relevant neurological signs, and the clinician should be prepared to discuss this with

Table 6.2 Investigations for depression in later life		
Investigation	First episode	Recurrence
Full blood count	Yes	Yes
Urea and electrolytes	Yes	Yes
Calcium	Yes	Yes
Thyroid function	Yes	If clinically indicated, or more than 12 months elapsed
B_{12}	Yes	If clinically indicated, or more than 12 months elapsed
Folate	Yes	If clinically indicated (e.g., recent poor diet)
Liver function	Yes	If indicated (e.g., suspected or known alcohol misuse)
Syphilitic serology	If clinically indicated (e.g., relevant neurological symptoms)	Only if clinically indicated
CT (brain)	If clinically indicated	If clinically indicated
EEG	If clinically indicated	If clinically indicated

the patient. The electroencephalogram (EEG) shows no specific changes in depression but can help differentiate it from dementia or delirium. Neuroimaging in affective disorders is done largely to rule out a space-occupying lesion and in treatment-resistant cases where vascular brain disease is suspected.

6.2.2 Assessment of executive function

There are a number of neuropsychological tests or test batteries which can point to executive cognitive problems. Verbal fluency (letter fluency and category naming) is a sensitive screening test of executive dysfunction in late-life depression (Alexopoulos 2005). Other 'bedside' tests can be carried out if the syndrome is suspected (Box 6.1). Examine the patient for a grasp reflex by gently scratching the inside of each palm looking for evidence of grasping. After demonstrating yourself, ask the patient to carry out the action of making a fist, then a cutting motion with the side of the hand and finally slapping palm downwards (known as the Luria motor sequencing task). The patient should be able to carry out three sequences in each hand smoothly. Draw a sequence of alternating squares and triangles using a single line and ask the patient to do the same; this degrades with frontal executive impairment. The Controlled Oral Word Association Test is a measure of self-monitoring, verbal fluency, categorization, and initiation. Ask the patient to generate as many words as he or she can think of with three different phonemic letter cues (most often F, A, and S or C, F, and L) each in a 60-second period. A total raw score of below 30 for patients aged 70 and above with less than 15 years of education suggests impairment. For animal naming, a score below 12 is suspicious (Gladsjo et al. 1999). However, educational attainment and ethnicity can affect scores, so they must be treated only as a guide.

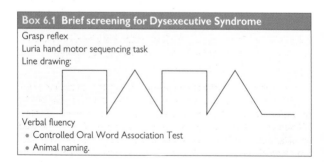

Box 6.1 Brief screening for Dysexecutive Syndrome
Grasp reflex
Luria hand motor sequencing task
Line drawing:
Verbal fluency
• Controlled Oral Word Association Test
• Animal naming.

6.3 **Pharmacotherapy**

6.3.1 **Pharmacological considerations in ageing**

The most important consideration is recognizing that inter-individual difference in drug handling is much greater in older than younger adults (Lotrich and Pollock 2005). Pharmacodynamic considerations include alterations in receptor numbers and affinity and in homeostatic mechanisms. Usually, this leads to increased sensitivity to various side effects at relatively low concentrations of antidepressants. An example is the higher risk of antimuscarinic side effects with tricyclic antidepressants (TCAs). Changes in pharmacodynamics may lead to impaired orthostatic responses, impaired thermoregulation, and a risk of delirium. However, altered pharmacodynamics may be responsible for a decrease in responsiveness to some drugs.

Pharmacokinetic response is affected by reduced renal clearance of the main and any active metabolites, diminished microsomal metabolism (involving the P450 systems), a smaller liver mass, reduced hepatic blood flow, and age-related decrements in total albumin and plasma binding. Genetic variation has also been shown to differentially affect the metabolism of antidepressants.

To put this knowledge base into practice, observe appropriate prescribing practice for older adults. Taylor et al. (2007) suggest the following: avoiding drugs which block α_1-adrenoreceptors, have antimuscarinic properties, are very sedative or markedly affect P450 enzyme systems (Table 6.7); start at low dose first; and try to minimize the number of drugs given and the number of times per day.

The management of depressive disorder is divided into three stages - see Chapter 9. Acute treatment refers to the period from initiation of treatment via improvement to remission. This usually covers a matter of weeks.

A number of studies indicate that psychotic depression requires treatment with both an antidepressant and an antipsychotic drug, or ECT. For older patients and antidepressants in particular, the adage 'start low—go slow' is apt. Prolonged dose titration is, however, usually unnecessary with most of the current antidepressants.

6.3.2 **Efficacy**

Two Cochrane systematic reviews of randomized controlled trials (RCTs) in later life can be summarized as follows. In the first review, compared to placebo, all antidepressants were more effective (Wilson et al. 2001). A second review (Mottram et al. 2006) showed no difference in efficacy between atypical antidepressants and selective serotonin reuptake inhibitors (SSRIs), but atypical antidepressants were associated with higher withdrawal rates due to side effects. Patients receiving tricyclic-related antidepressants (Mianserin or Trazodone) had a similar withdrawal rate to SSRIs, suggesting that tricyclic-related antidepressants may offer a viable alternative to SSRIs in older depressed patients. Mirtazapine, too new for these reviews, can probably be included in this category by inference, venlafaxine acts like an SSRI, and there are data on older adults showing efficacy for duloxetine. A caution though is that in many recent clinical trials of antidepressants across all age groups, remission rates are much lower than response rates. This may be because some trials are too short, often only 4–6 weeks, for full efficacy to be demonstrated or that the 'placebo' response is much higher than is generally thought (see later).

6.3.3 Starting treatment

6.3.3.1 Consent and capacity

It is important to check and record that the patient understands the proposed treatment and agrees to it. Details about mental capacity and its assessment are beyond the scope of this book. In England, a new Mental Capacity Act (2005) has set the legal framework. Information is available on the Department of Constitutional Affairs website (http://www.dca.gov.uk/menincap/legis.htm). A summary of key points is listed in Box 6.2. Patients with severe depression or depression with dementia may have to be treated under this legal framework if it is in the person's best interests. Involvement with caregivers and relatives is important but unless the patient lacks mental capacity and it is in their best interests, this should always be with the patient's permission.

Box 6.2 Principles and guidance about capacity assessments from Mental Capacity Act (2005) in England

- Assume a person has capacity unless proved otherwise
- Do not treat people as incapable of making a decision unless you have tried all you can to help them
- Do not treat someone as incapable of making a decision because their decision may seem unwise
- Do things or take decisions for people without capacity in their best interests
- Before doing something to someone or making a decision on their behalf, consider whether you could achieve the outcome in a less restrictive way
- Be clear about the decision to be made and who is the decision-maker
- The key principle is that all decisions must be made in the best interests of the person who lacks capacity, taking into consideration all relevant circumstances
- The Act does not define best interests but does give a checklist:
  - Must involve the person who lacks capacity
  - Have regard for past and present wishes and feelings
  - Consult with others who are involved in the care of the person
  - Undertake the assessment under circumstances which maximize the person's capabilities
  - Document the decision and review it as necessary

In England from April 2009 an amendment to the Mental Capacity Act (2005) means that new procedures must be adopted for incapacitous persons whose best interests can only be met via interventions in a hospital or registered care home which lead to them being deprived of their liberty. The relevant website is http://www.dh.gov.uk/en/SocialCare/Deliveringadultsocialcare/MentalCapacity/MentalCapacityActDeprivationofLibertySafeguards/DH_084948.

Again it is possible that some severely depressed patients and some patients with depression complicating dementia or another organic brain syndrome could be affected.

Mental Health legislation exists for patients who because of their disordered state of mind (which may include severe depression) refuse treatment that will prevent harm to themselves, others, or will avoid catastrophic deterioration in their health. In England, this is the 2007 Mental Health Act (http://www.opsi.gov.uk/acts/acts2007/ukpga_20070012_en_1).

6.3.3.2 Discussion with the patient

Patients worry that antidepressants are addictive, and that depression is 'senility' or an inevitable sign of dementia. Reassurance and encouragement to stick with the treatment is important; the patient must be helped to understand that results take time, otherwise they will give up early in treatment. Goals of treatment should be discussed and agreed with the patient (Baldwin et al. 2002). Commonly occurring side effects should be explained.

There is a high placebo response rate in controlled trials of antidepressants. This is probably because placebo treatment involves much more than a pill. In scientific trials to establish the efficacy of a compound, participants will see members of the research team who may provide empathic listening and informal support. These 'non-specific' factors in the treatment of late-life depressive disorder are nowadays widely recognized as a key component of care. Probable components include having a plausible treatment delivered by someone perceived as an expert who is enthusiastic about it and takes depression seriously; the expectation of improvement; the positive regard of the prescriber towards the patient; listening with empathy; encouraging verbalization of distress; and, perhaps especially important in older adults, encouragement to undertake purposeful activity to counter apathy and withdrawal.

Building the therapeutic relationship in this way is important in establishing treatment concordance. Not taking medication is the major cause of treatment failure. Box 6.3 lists key aspects of concordance to consider.

6.4 Pharmacological management in the acute phase

6.4.1 Classification of antidepressant used to treat older adults

A classification of antidepressants is shown in Box 6.4.

Box 6.3 Practical aspects of concordance in treatment

- Understanding the patient's perception of what depression is and that of his/her family and supporters
- Explaining what depression is and what it is not (e.g., 'weakness of character')
- Clarifying attribution of symptoms (e.g., all due to heart, bowels, etc.)
- Explaining side effects
- Explaining delay in onset
- Agreeing management plan and treatment goals involving family/supporters with consent of the patient

---

Box 6.4 Classification of antidepressants

Older tricyclics
Secondary amines (nortriptyline)
Tertiary amines (imipramine, amitriptyline, dosulepin (dothiepin), clomipramine)
Newer tricyclics
Lofepramine
Atypical antidepressants
Trazodone, mianserin
Monoamine oxidase inhibitors (non-reversible)
Phenelzine, tranylcypromine
Reversible inhibitors of monoamine oxidase A ('RIMA' agents)
Moclobemide
Selective serotonin reuptake inhibitors (SSRIs)
Fluvoxamine, fluoxetine, paroxetine, sertraline, citalopram, escitalopram
Noradrenaline and specific serotonin enhancers (NASSa)
Mirtazapine
Noradrenaline reuptake inihibitors (NARIs)
Reboxetine*
Serotonin/noradrenaline reuptake inhibitors (SNRIs)
Venlafaxine
Duloxetine

*Not recommended for older adults in the United Kingdom because of lack of evidence at the time of granting a license.

6.4.2 Individual drugs and dosages

The main mode of action of antidepressants and the average starting and therapeutic dosages are listed in Table 6.3. With so many antidepressants to choose from the principle is to match the antidepressant to the patient, taking into account tolerability, safety, likely side effects, drug interactions, and contraindications. The three most commonly prescribed SSRIs, citalopram, sertraline, and escitalopram, are non-sedative whereas mirtazapine is sedative and may be helpful for depression-associated insomnia.

Table 6.3 Mode of action, side effect profiles, and dosages of main antidepressants used to treat late-life depression in the United Kingdom (see also Baldwin et al. 2002; Unutzer 2007)

Drug	Main mode of action	Main side effects	Starting dosage (mg)	Average daily dose (mg)
Amitriptyline	NA^{++} $5\text{-}HT^+$	Sedation antimuscarinic, postural hypotension, tachycardia/arrhythmia	25–50	75–100*
Imipramine	NA^{++} $5\text{-}HT^+$	As for amitriptyline but less sedation	25	75–100*
Nortriptyline	NA^{++} $5\text{-}HT^+$	As for amitriptyline but less sedation, antimuscarinic effects, and hypotension	10 tds	75–100*
Dothiepin	NA^{++} $5\text{-}HT^+$	As for amitriptyline	50–75	75–150*
Mianserin	α_2	Sedation	30	30–90
Lofepramine	NA^{++} $5\text{-}HT^+$	As for amitriptyline but less sedation, antimuscarinic effects, hypotension, and cardiac problems	70–140	70–210
Trazodone	$5\text{-}HT_2$	Sedation, dizziness, headache	100	300
Citalopram	$5\text{-}HT$	Nausea, vomiting, dyspepsia, abdominal pain, diarrhoea, headache, sexual dysfunction; risk of gastric bleeding; inappropriate ADH secretion	20	20–40
Sertraline	$5\text{-}HT$	As for citalopram	50	50–150

Table 6.3 *Contd.*

Drug	Main mode of action	Main side effects	Starting dosage (mg)	Average daily dose (mg)
Fluoxetine	5-HT	As for citalopram but insomnia and agitation more common	20	20*
Paroxetine	5-HT	As for citalopram but sedation and anticholinergic effects may occur	20	20
Fluvoxamine	5-HT	As for citalopram but nausea more common	50–100	100–200
Escitalopram	5-HT	As for citalopram	5	10
Moclobemide	MAO	Sleep disturbance, nausea, agitation	300	300–400
Venlafaxine	NA 5-HT	Nausea, insomnia, dizziness, dry mouth, somnolence, hyper- and hypotension	75	150**
Duloxetine	NA 5-HT	Nausea, insomnia, dizziness	30	60–90
Mirtazapine	α_2 blocking selective antagonist 5-HT$_2$ and 5-HT$_3$ receptors	Increased appetite, weight gain, somnolence, headache	15	30–45

NA = noradrenaline; 5-HT = serotonin; MAO = monoamine oxidase.

* These are average doses. Some patients will require higher dosages depending on response and tolerability.

** Titration up to higher dosages is common in specialist care.

⁺Indicates relative strength of monoamine effect.

6.4.3 Side effects and interactions

The P450 enzyme systems are the main mode of metabolism. Via the 2D6 system, prescription of SSRIs such as paroxetine and fluoxetine and the dual-acting drug duloxetine can lead to inhibition of the metabolism of TCAs, antipsychotics, lipophilic β-blockers, some analgesics (such as codeine), some antiarrhythmics, and triazolobenzodiazepines, such as alprazolam. Adverse interactions between SSRIs and TCAs occur because each may inhibit the metabolism of the other. Via the 2C and 3A enzyme systems, fluoxetine and paroxetine can inhibit the metabolism of benzodiazepines, calcium channel blockers, and theophylline and enhance the effects of phenytoin. Table 6.4 shows that citalopram, escitalopram,

Table 6.4 Inhibition of P450 enzymes by SSRIs (see also Taylor et al. 2007)

Enzyme group inhibited by SSRI	IA2	2C9	2D6	3A
Example of substrate	Caffeine	Phenytoin	Tricyclics	Benzodiazepines
Fluoxetine	+	++	+++	++
Sertraline	+	+	+	+
Paroxetine	+	+	+++	+
Citalopram	+	0	+	0
Escitalopram	0	0	0	0
Fluvoxamine	+++	++	+	++

Degree of inhibition: 0 = minimal; + = mild inhibition; ++ = moderate inhibition; +++ = strong inhibition.

and sertraline are least likely of the SSRIs to be involved in P450 interactions and are therefore often recommended as first-line antidepressants in late-life depression. Venlafaxine acts like an SSRI with minimal effects on the 2D6 enzyme. Mirtazapine too has minimal effects on 1A2, C9, and 2D6.

Table 6.3 shows the main side effects of antidepressants used to treat late-life depression. Antimuscarinic side effects include dry mouth, blurred vision, constipation, and urinary retention and are common with TCA treatment. Cardiotoxicity is a further concern and it is recommended that an electrocardiogram (ECG) be carried out before commencing an older TCA. Cardiac arrhythmia in TCA overdose can be fatal. In medically unwell patients delirium can occur. Postural hypotension due to adrenergic blockade is a serious problem with TCAs and dual-acting drugs (SNRIs). With the TCAs and mirtazapine, histaminic effects can cause sedation and weight gain. Lofepramine is a second generation TCA less likely to cause these adverse effects.

SSRIs are safer than TCAs but they have their own side effects, including nausea (around 15%), diarrhoea (around 10%), insomnia (5%–15%), anxiety and/or agitation (2%–15%), headache, weight loss, and sexual dysfunction (an area hardly ever inquired of with older people, hence its prevalence is almost certainly underestimated). SSRIs have minimal impact on cognitive function in older patients with depression and may have less impairment on driving skills than older drugs. Because SSRIs are associated with bleeding risk, gastroprotective medication is recommended for older patients on non-steroidal anti-inflammatory drugs (NSAIDs) or aspirin or a prior history of ulcer or bleeding problems (Table 6.5). There are also concerns that SSRIs may lower bone density through their effects on serotonin transporter in bone tissue (Haney and Warden 2009). To what extent this is clinically relevant is not yet clear although reports are beginning to appear of increased falls and hip fracture in patients taking SSRIs (Richards et al. 2007).

53

- Delirium
- Postural hypotension
- Gastric bleeding
- Inappropriate ADH (IADH) secretion
- Falls and/or unsteadiness

After 4 weeks of treatment, discontinuation symptoms may occur if the antidepressant is stopped suddenly. This is more likely with short half-life drugs (and therefore least likely with fluoxetine) and particularly likely with paroxetine and venlafaxine. SSRIs may cause inappropriate antidiuretic hormone (IADH) secretion; and increased age, female gender, and drugs that lower sodium levels are all risk factors. Symptoms of IADH, which include lethargy, fatigue, and sleep disturbance, as well as muscle cramps and headaches, overlap with those of depression.

Moclobemide is well tolerated by older people and although a special diet is not required, patients should be aware of the drug interactions with painkillers and other antidepressants. Co-prescriptions of moclobemide with tricyclics or SSRIs should be avoided. A washout period of around 4–5 half-lives of the drug and any active metabolite is advised when transferring from a tricyclic or SSRI to moclobemide (but is not necessary from moclobemide to a tricyclic or SSRI).

Venlafaxine is generally well tolerated provided the dose is increased incrementally. Hypertension is a known problem with venlafaxine but in older patients postural hypotension can also occur (Table 6.4.3). Venlafaxine is not recommended in patients with heart disease likely to predispose to arrhythmia. Duloxetine, a newer dual-acting antidepressant, has not been shown to be cardiotoxic.

Of other drugs, mirtazapine and trazodone have similar side effects to TCAs, including urinary retention in older men. There are occasional reports of priapism with trazodone. Concerns over blood dyscrasias necessitating regular blood counts make mianserin inconvenient to use.

6.5 Next steps for patients not responsive to treatment

In a recent meta-analysis of randomized trials involving newer antidepressants the mean period response rates for antidepressants response was 44.4% (Nelson *et al.* 2006). Therefore a high percentage of patients will not recover with the first antidepressants prescribed. Box 6.6 shows a strategy to follow before the patient is considered 'resistant' to treatment. Although it is often stated that older patients take longer to recover this is less true with the advent of newer antidepressants, so that failure of response at 4 weeks should prompt a review of

> **Box 6.6 Strategy for non-responsive patients**
>
> (1) If little or no response (<25% reduction in symptoms) by 4 weeks:
> - Increase the dose OR if dosage optimal, change antidepressants (Rush 2007) either within SSRI or to a different class (Anderson *et al*, 2008)
>
> (2) If partial response by 4 weeks:
> - Optimize dose (if not already done)
> - Continue and review 2–4 weekly
>
> (3) If little further improvement by 8 weeks:
> - Consider augmentation, either with medication or a psychological intervention (but seek specialist advice regarding medication)
>
> OR
> - Consider combining antidepressants (but seek specialist advice)
>
> (4) At all stages consider electroconvulsive therapy if indicated by severity or risks

> **Box 6.7 A systematic approach to resistant depression**
>
> - Review the diagnosis (e.g., is this psychotic depression?)
> - Review treatment adequacy (duration, dose, compliance)
> - Ensure that a logical framework has been used (rational sequential treatment ('stepped care') within a framework or protocol)
> - Measure outcome appropriately (e.g., symptoms of depression and social recovery from depression may follow different trajectories)
> - Address medical co-morbidity (note in late-onset cases consider vascular depression)
> - Address psychiatric morbidity (e.g., residual anxiety, insomnia)
> - Consider factors in the treatment setting including family and relationship factors that have been overlooked (e.g., avoidance behaviour and overdependency)

treatment, provided the dosage is optimum. Prolonging the treatment period is only realistic for patients who have begun to respond.

Box 6.7 shows what to look for before concluding that the patient is 'resistant' to treatment.

6.6 Resistant depression

There is no universally agreed guideline as to what constitutes resistance to treatment. If there is genuine non-response after two trials of different antidepressants each of at least four weeks duration at optimal dosaging (after the higher end of the recommended range) then there are a number of strategies (Table 6.5) to consider. Persistence pays. In a clinical series, Flint and Rifat (1996) using a rational sequential (stepped care) protocol showed that sequential regimes of antidepressant therapy eventually produced improvement or recovery in over 80% of their patients.

6.6.1 Combining antidepressants

Dodd *et al.* (2005) conducted a literature review (not specific to older patients) on combining antidepressants and suggested that combination treatment helps about 50% of patients not responsive to antidepressant monotherapy. Although generally safe, some adverse reactions were reported, including one report of the serotonergic syndrome (Box 6.8). For older patients, there are little specific data and we are reliant on extrapolating from this broader research, always remembering that older patients are more susceptible to adverse effects and drug interactions. Popular combinations include an SSRI plus mirtazapine, an SSRI plus venlafaxine, and venlafaxine plus mirtazapine, but these should only be undertaken by specialists.

6.6.2 Augmentation

Although its use has waned in recent years, lithium augmentation remains an effective treatment for the management of resistant depression. Its use can be difficult in older patients as side effects and the risk of toxicity are higher. Side effects affecting a quarter or more of older adults on lithium are polydipsia, polyuria, mild tremor, dry mouth, nausea, and memory impairment. Toxicity (marked tremor, unsteadiness, incoordination, confusion, and altered level of consciousness)

Table 6.5 Strategies for resistant depression	
Strategy	**Example**
Optimization (Maximize dose/serum level/time)	• Dose increase • Prolong course • Measure/adjust drug concentration (tricyclics only)
Substitution (Substitute one antidepressant for another)	• SSRI to SSRI • SSRI to a different class
Augmentation (Use of a non-primary antidepressant)	• Lithium • Atypical antipsychotic • Psychological intervention • Triiodothyronine (T3)
Combination (Use two primary antidepressants together)	• SSRI + mirtazapine • Mirtazapine + venlafaxine • SSRI + bupropion

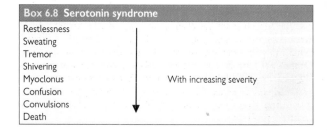

Box 6.8 Serotonin syndrome	
Restlessness Sweating Tremor Shivering Myoclonus Confusion Convulsions Death	With increasing severity

may affect 10% of older patients at some point during lithium treatment. The risk is increased by dehydration such as caused by a chest infection, other febrile illness, or diarrhoea and vomiting. Renal disease is another risk factor as is treatment with diuretics and NSAIDs. Do not forget that lithium toxicity has been reported in patients with brain damage even at serum levels in the therapeutic range; the clinical picture is the best guide. A safer option may be augmentation with L triiodothyronine (T3) at dosages of between 25–30 mg although there are no data concerning older adults and excessive thyroid supplementation can strain the heart.

Some geriatric psychiatrists suggest using low dosage lithium, aiming for a serum level of around 0.35–0.5mmol/L instead of the current recommended one of 0.6–0.8mmol/L for new patients (NICE 2006). This may be appropriate for the prophylaxis of depression and bipolar disorder but possibly not for lithium augmentation in depressive disorder. A recent study by Kok and colleagues (2008) investigated the outcome of a sequential treatment protocol in older patients not responding to a 12-week trial comprising venlafaxine versus nortriptyline. Of 81 patients, 78 achieved a response and 68 (84%) entered remission within three years of treatment. Twenty-two patients received lithium with a remission rate of two thirds, higher than some other recent studies of lithium augmentation but the mean lithium level was 0.82mmol/L. The recommendation then is to treat to the higher range if tolerated.

Although there are limited data specific to older patients, there is growing evidence that augmentation of antidepressants with atypical antipsychotic medication is effective and may help target symptoms such as anxiety and agitation. In the United States, aripiprazole has a license for resistant depression.

Psychological interventions (discussed later) should be considered as valid strategies for augmentation of antidepressants. Do not forget exercise is an antidepressant.

6.6.3 Electroconvulsive therapy

Similar to lithium, the use of ECT has declined but less so for older adults, perhaps because it is effective and often better tolerated than multiple medications. Opinion is divided about bilateral versus unilateral delivery of ECT. Traditionally, bilateral ECT has been regarded as more effective than unilateral but research with high dosage unilateral ECT shows remission rates as good as bilateral. However, increasing the dose causes more cognitive impairment and this is the major risk for older adults. A compromise is to start with unilateral placement and continue with bilateral if there has been no response after 4–6 treatments.

Headache and memory loss are the most commonly reported side effects. The latter causes amnesia particularly at the time of the administration of ECT.

An important drawback with ECT is the high subsequent relapse rate and how to avoid this. The best evidence suggests giving an antidepressant plus lithium, but probably also the new generation antipsychotics to prevent relapse. Because depression in later life is associated with an increased chance of relapse, there may be a place for maintenance ECT, often given fortnightly or monthly.

6.6.4 **Other strategies**

Because of dietary restrictions, traditional monoamine oxidase inhibitors (MAOIs) are rarely used although there were some early reports of success.

L-Tryptophan may have a role as an adjunctive therapy in treatment-resistant depression but has been associated with the eosinophilic myalgia syndrome and a risk of the serotonin syndrome when combined with other antidepressants such as SSRIs (Box 6.8).

The main role for anticonvulsants in depression is lamotrigine for bipolar depression. Pregabalin, licensed for generalized anxiety disorder, has been shown to be effective in older adults (Montgomery et al. 2008). Since residual anxiety is a common intractable problem in treating older adults, the use of this drug adjunctively may have a place in resistant depression.

Repetitive transcranial magnetic stimulation (rTMS) is a reasonably effective treatment for moderate depressive episode but there have been no adequate RCTs in older patients. Frontal atrophy, as can occur in late-life vascular depression, may reduce the response to rTMS in older patients. Jorge et al. (2008) studied rTMS in 92 patients with major depression aged over 50 with vascular depression randomized to rTMS (12,000 pulses), rTMS (18,000 pulses), or sham rTMS, over a 10-day period. Using the 18k paradigm, there was a significantly better response in the actively treated group although remission rates were fairly low in all three groups. Age predicted a poorer response. Volume of white matter disease was not a predictor of response but lower frontal gray matter volume was.

Vagal Nerve Stimulation is a novel treatment for resistant depression although no efficacy or tolerability data exist for older adults. Finally, psychosurgery is still used in a few designated centres. Success is reported, although the patients referred to these centres are usually middle aged rather than elderly.

6.7 **Treatment in special situations**

6.7.1 **Depression in dementia**

The principles of treating depression associated with dementia are no different from those of 'uncomplicated' depression but with the caveat that spontaneous recovery ('placebo response') often occurs, so that watchful waiting is justified. Few good clinical studies have been conducted although the current recommendation is to treat with an SSRI. An unanswered question is whether antidepressant treatment may improve not only depression but also cognitive impairment.

6.7.2 Stroke

As with dementia, spontaneous recovery from depression occurs after stroke but is less likely as time goes by. Research suggests it is particularly unlikely after six weeks.

A recent review of the literature found only 10 RCTs of antidepressants (fluoxetine, citalopram, sertraline, nortriptyline) in post-stroke depression. There was evidence of efficacy but the quality and size of the trials was variable (Paranthaman and Baldwin 2006). Stimulants such as methylphenidate 5–10mg daily may benefit stroke-related apathy but they are not recommended for routine use and are unlicensed for this indication.

There is little evidence for the efficacy of psychological interventions in post-stroke depression but this is largely because such studies are difficult to conduct.

Both TCAs and SSRIs are effective in treating emotionalism. There are also reports of the successful use of mirtazapine and venlafaxine. SSRIs are currently the recommended first-line treatment on grounds of reduced side effects (Paranthaman and Baldwin 2006). Unlike depression, a response is often seen within the first week, irrespective of lesion location or time since stroke.

Small studies are beginning to suggest that rTMS is effective in post-stroke depression, although this treatment is not widely available.

6.7.3 Coronary heart disease

Treatment of depression with an antidepressant or a psychological intervention produces only modest improvements in depression, and no study to date has shown clear benefits of treatment for coronary heart disease (CHD) morbidity and mortality. However, because SSRIs decrease platelet function, there is a theoretical reason for thinking that SSRI treatment may reduce cardiac mortality (Evans et al. 2005).

Tricyclic antidepressants are type 1A antiarrhythmics and they can reduce heart rate variability, a factor linked to increased mortality. There is no evidence to implicate SSRIs in adversely affecting cardiac function. Venlafaxine can increase blood pressure, although in older patients it can cause postural hypotension. It should not be used in patients with a significant risk of ventricular arrhythmia. Lithium treatment can potentiate arrhythmia and has been linked to heart block. Therefore, the current recommended treatment for depression following an acute cardiac event or with stable heart disease is an SSRI.

6.7.4 Diabetes

Depression in diabetes is usually treated with an SSRI. TCAs are more likely to impair diabetic control than SSRIs, although fluoxetine should be used with caution as it can cause hypoglycaemia. TCAs can help painful neuropathy. Mirtazapine may cause weight gain (a risk factor for diabetes), lithium toxicity is increased if there is nephropathy, and valproate may give a false positive result on urine testing for glucose. There is also interest in the use of alternative and complementary medicine to improve glycaemic control and mood in diabetic patients. These include Ayurvedic medicine, exercise, mindfulness, yoga, and acupuncture. There is also some evidence of benefits from cognitive behavioural therapy (CBT). However, as with the treatment of depression in heart disease, it is yet to be demonstrated that interventions are disease-modifying (as measured by glycosylated haemoglobin levels).

6.7.5 Parkinson's disease

L-DOPA does not seem to improve mood in the patients of Parkinson's disease. Serotonin and noradrenaline systems are probably more important and usually SSRIs are given because tricyclics aggravate constipation and postural hypotension, as well as increasing confusion via antimuscarinic effects. However, there are few well-controlled clinical trials for the treatment of depression in Parkinson's disease, and a recent study of patients with a mean age of 62 years showed that nortriptyline, a TCA, was more effective than controlled release paroxetine as well as being well tolerated (Menza et al. 2009). Concerns have been expressed that SSRIs can cause emergent extrapyramidal effects but this is controversial. The combination of an SSRI and selegilene can lead to the potentially fatal serotonin syndrome (Box 6.8).

Tianeptine (which increases the presynaptic recapture of 5-hydroxy indoleacetic acid) and moclobemide (a reversible and selective inhibitor of monoamine oxidase) have been used to treat depression in Parkinson's disease, but the evidence is largely empirical and tianeptine is marketed worldwide. Deep brain stimulation is a treatment for both Parkinson's disease and severe depression although paradoxically it may provoke depression in Parkinson's patients.

Electroconvulsive therapy is effective in treating severe depression with Parkinson's disease and improving motor symptoms, albeit temporarily. There are some studies of rTMS in depression associated with Parkinson's disease and further evidence is awaited.

6.7.6 Chronic obstructive pulmonary disease

There are no high-quality trials of antidepressants in chronic obstructive pulmonary disease (COPD), but given the association of COPD depression with anxiety symptoms, an SSRI or mirtazapine can be given. Benzodiazepines should be avoided as they depress respiration. Pulmonary rehabilitation based on activation and physical conditioning along with an antidepressant may be an effective approach compared with medication alone. CBT and group educational interventions have been found to alleviate depression and anxiety symptoms and improve quality of life in patients with COPD (Kunik et al. 2007).

6.7.7 **Pain**

Where depression and pain coexist, treatment with both analgesics and antidepressants leads to better depression outcomes and lower reported pain than either given alone.

6.8 **Psychological treatments**

Age is no barrier to psychological interventions for depression; for moderate depressive disorder they are as effective as medication (Pinquart et al. 2006). Currently, there is evidence for the efficacy of CBT and behaviour therapy, interpersonal therapy (IPT), and dynamic psychotherapy. Most research though has been conducted using CBT and IPT. CBT helps the patient in the here and now to understand the links between low mood and both negative cognitions and behaviour. In IPT, the emphasis is on current problems within the interpersonal context. An understanding of past relationships may help but is not a major emphasis. IPT aims to help patients change, rather than to simply understand and accept their current life situation.

Problem Solving Treatment (PST) is of proven efficacy in younger patients with mild-to-moderate depression. PST also deals with the here and now, focusing on current difficulties and setting future goals. It is designed to help the patient gain a sense of mastery over difficulties.

It is based on CBT principles but unlike CBT requires less training and can be taught to non-psychiatrically trained health professionals. As such, it offers promise in the treatment of older people with depressive disorder. There is a drawback to its simplicity. One research trial show that efficacy varied greatly across participating sites because efficacy depended on the skills of therapist: more experienced therapists got better results (Williams et al. 2000). Although less widely available, CBT training is more in depth and the training is more standardized.

Of those studies which have compared antidepressants drugs with psychotherapies and with combined treatments, the combination appears to be more effective than either given alone, and the effect appears stronger in patients with more severe depression. Importantly, this appears to be so in older patients even where there is a clear trigger such as bereavement (Reynolds et al. 1999).

It is sometimes necessary to modify techniques such as CBT with older adults but the modifications required are not as extensive as is sometimes supposed—older adults adapt well to this approach. Common sense changes include repetition, writing things down, and shorter sessions.

Family therapy has been adapted for use with older patients and there are case reports of its efficacy in both dementia and depression. In a RCT, a family intervention delivered to carers of patients with dementia resulted in significant reduction of stress, burden, and depressive symptoms, with a number needed to treat of two (Marriott *et al.* 2000).

Key references

Alexopoulos GS (2005). Depression in the elderly. *The Lancet*, **365**(9475), 1961–70.

Anderson IM, Ferrier IN, Baldwin R, *et al.* (2008). Evidence-based guidelines for treating depressive disorders based guidelines for treating depressive disorders with antidepressants: A revision of the 2000 British Association for Psychopharmacology guidelines *Journal of Psychopharmacology*, **22**, 343–96.

Baldwin RC, Chiu E, Katona C, and Graham N (2002). *Guidelines on depression in older people: practising the evidence.* Under the auspices of the World Psychiatric Association Sections of Old Age Psychiatry and Affective Disorders. Martin Dunitz, London.

Brooke P and Bullock R (1999). Validation of the 6 Item Cognitive Impairment Test. *International Journal of Geriatric Psychiatry*, **14**, 936–40.

Dodd S, Horgan D, Malhi GS, and Berk M (2005). To combine or not to combine? A literature review of antidepressant combination therapy. *Journal of Affective Disorders*, **89**(1–3), 1–11.

Evans DL, Charney DS, Lewis L, *et al.* (2005). Mood disorders in the medically Ill: scientific review and recommendations *Biological Psychiatry*, **58**, 175–89.

Flint AJ and Rifat SL (1996). The effect of sequential antidepressant treatment on geriatric depression. Journal of Affective Disorders, 36, 95–105.

Folstein MF, Folstein SE, and McHugh PR (1975). "Mini-Mental State": a practical method for grading the cognitive state of patients for the clinician Journal of Psychiatric Research, 12, 185–98.

Gladsjo JA, Schuman CC, Evans JD, Peavy GM, Miller GW, and Heaton RK (1999). Norms for letter and category fluency: demographic corrections for age, education, and ethnicity. *Assessment*, **6**, 147–78.

Haney EM and Warden SJ (2009). Skeletal effects of serotonin (5-hydroxytryptamine) transporter inhibition: evidence from clinical studies. *Journal of Musculoskeletal and Neuronal Interactions*, **8**, 133–45.

Jorge JRE, Moser DJ, Acion L, and Robinson RG (2008). Treatment of vascular depression using repetitive transcranial magnetic stimulation. *Archives of General Psychiatry*, **65**, 268–76.

Kok RM, Nolen WA, and Heeren TJ (2009). Outcome of late-life depression after 3 years of sequential treatment. *Acta Psychiatrica Scandinavica*, **119**, 274–81.

Kunik ME, Veazey C, Cully JA, et al. (2007). COPD education and cognitive behavioural therapy group treatment for clinically significant symptoms of depression and anxiety in COPD patients: a randomized controlled trial. *Psychological Medicine*, **37**, 1–12.

Lotrich FE and Pollock BG (2005). Aging and clinical pharmacology: implications for antidepressants. *Journal of Clinical Pharmacology*, **45**, 1106–22.

Marriott A, Donaldson C, Tarrier N, and Burns A (2000). Effectiveness of cognitive-behavioural family intervention in reducing the burden of care in carers of patients with Alzheimer's disease. *British Journal of Psychiatry*, **176**, 557–62.

Menza M, Dobkin RD, Marin H, et al. (2009). A controlled trial of antidepressants in patients with Parkinson disease and depression. *Neurology*, **72**, 886–92.

Montgomery S, Chatamra K, Pauer L, Whalen E, and Baldinetti F (2008). Efficacy and safety of pregabalin in elderly people with generalised anxiety disorder. *British Journal of Psychiatry*, **193**, 389–94.

Mottram P, Wilson K, and Strobl J (2006). Antidepressants for depressed elderly. *The Cochrane Database of Systematic Reviews*, Issue 1.

National Institute for Health and Clinical Excellence (NICE) (2004). Depression: management of depression in primary and secondary care (Clinical guideline 23). NICE, London.

National Institute for Health and Clinical Excellence (NICE) (2006). Bipolar disorder. The management of bipolar disorder in adults, children and adolescent in primary and secondary care. NICE cilnical guidance 38.

Nelson JC, Delucchi K, Schneider LS (2008). Efficacy of second generation antidepressants in late-life depression: a meta-analysis of the evidence. *American Journal of Geriatric Psychiatry*, **16**, 558–67.

Paranthaman R and Baldwin RC (2006). Treatments of psychiatric syndromes due to cerebrovascular disease. *International Review of Psychiatry*, **18**(5), 453–70.

Pinquart M, Duberstein PR, and Lyness JM (2006). Treatments for later-life depressive conditions: a meta-analytic comparison of pharmacotherapy and psychotherapy. *American Journal of Psychiatry*, **163**(9), 1493–501.

Reynolds CF III, Frank E, Perel JM, et al. (1999). Nortriptyline and interpersonal psychotherapy as maintenance therapies for recurrent major depression: a randomized controlled trial in patients older then 59 years. *Journal of the American Medical Association*, **281**, 39–45.

Richards JB, Papaioannou A, Adachi JD, for the Canadian Multicentre Osteoporosis Study (CaMos) Research Group 9 (2007). Effect of selective serotonin reuptake inhibitors on the risk of fracture. *Archives of Internal Medicine*, **167**, 188–94.

Rush AJ (2007). STAR* D: What Have We Learned? *Americal Journal of Psychiatry*, **164**, 201–40.

Taylor D, Paton C, and Kerwin R (2007). *The Maudsley prescribing guidelines*, 9th edn. Informa Health care, London.

Williams JW, Barrett J, Oxman T, *et al.* (2000). Treatment of dysthymia and minor depression in primary care: a randomised controlled trial in older adults. *JAMA*, **284**, 1519–26.

Wilson K, Mottram P, Sivanranthan A, and Nightingale A (2001). Antidepressant versus placebo for depressed elderly (Cochrane Review). *The Cochrane Database of Systematic Reviews*, Issue 2, CD000561.

Chapter 7

Depression in primary care

> **Key points**
>
> - There are several instruments which can be used to screen older people for depression, including those with dementia plus depression.
> - Screening is most effective when targeted to those at most risk, factors which can be ascertained in older adults.
> - Most suicides in older adults have had recent contact with primary care services.
> - There are important barriers which must be overcome for the successful detection and management of depression in later life.
> - Collaborative care between primary and specialist care utilizing a depression care manager is more effective than usual care.

This chapter utilizes concepts and information from other chapters and adapts them to the context of primary care. Specialists (who in fact see only a small proportion of older depressed patients) often complain that depression in primary care is under-recognized and under-treated. Given the difficulties in diagnosing late-life depression and the arbitrary rule about when to offer antidepressant treatment, it is not surprising that primary care physicians find this a difficult area. Nevertheless, frequent presentation in a patient in primary care is one marker for possible depression in later life (Katona and Shankar 2004) so that primary care has a crucial role in the detection and treatment of late-life depressive disorder.

7.1 Detection and screening for depression

There is no evidence that 'universal' screening for depression in primary care improves outcomes. The chronic disease model, widely adopted in the UK primary care sector, suggests a different approach, targeted screening. For example, as mentioned, epidemiological data suggest that frequent attenders at primary care and those who have a high level of home care services are at risk of depression; they might be preferentially screened. In England, primary care practices pursuing the Quality and Outcomes Framework (QoF) of the General Practitioner (GP) contract have to screen patients for depression who have coronary heart disease (CHD) or diabetes (Quality Indicator DEP1) (BMA 2006). Other chronic illnesses such as chronic obstructive pulmonary disease (COPD) may be included in the future. Practices undertaking the National Enhanced Service for specialized care of patients with depression will be proactive in seeking cases and screening for them using recognized tools (Box 7.1 and Appendix).

The English National Institute for Health and Clinical Excellence (NICE) recommends a two-question screen for depression (Box 7.2). However, although it has high sensitivity (almost 100%), this short screen has low specificity and a recent review (Mitchell and Coyne 2007) suggests that ultra-short screening tests for depression are not sufficiently accurate for use in general practice.

The Geriatric Depression Scale (GDS) has been developed specifically for older adults. It has 30 questions and is reproduced in the Appendix. It avoids questions that rely on physical symptoms and uses a simple yes/no format. It is meant to be self-administered but rater assistance is acceptable. There are shorter versions, including a 15-item version and a 4-item one, using questions 1, 3, 8, and 9 (Box 7.3). There is a GDS website with various versions, bibliography, and translations into Chinese, Creole, Danish, Dutch,

> **Box 7.1 Screening instruments for late-life depression (see Appendix)**
>
> - Geriatric Depression Scale (GDS)
> - Hospital Anxiety and Depression Scale (HADS)
> - Patient Health Questionnaire (PHQ-9)
> - World Health Organization Well-Being Index
> - Cornell Scale for Depression in Dementia
>
> From NICE (2004).

> **Box 7.2 NICE Screening Questions for depression**
>
> - During the last month have you been feeling down, depressed, or hopeless?
> - During the last month have you often been bothered by having little interest or pleasure in doing things?

> **Box 7.3 The four most sensitive questions from the GDS[a]**
>
> - Are you basically satisfied with your life?
> - Do you feel that your life is empty?
> - Are you afraid that something bad is going to happen to you?
> - Do you feel happy most of the time?
>
> [a] A score of 2 or more indicates a probable depressive disorder.

Farsi, French, French Canadian, German, Greek, Hebrew, Hindi, Hungarian, Icelandic, Italian, Japanese, Korean, Lithuanian, Malay, Portuguese, Russian, Russian Ukrainian, Spanish, Swedish, Thai, Turkish, Vietnamese, and Yiddish (http://stanford.edu/~yesavage/GDS.html).

Despite its name, the Hospital Anxiety and Depression Scale (HADS) is also recommended for use in primary care and has been validated on older adults (Spinhoven *et al.* 1997). For screening in primary care, it is the total score which best predicts the likelihood of depression. It takes about 5 minutes to complete and its scores can be categorized as normal (0–7), mild (8–10), moderate (11–14), and severe (15–21), although research (Spinhoven *et al.* 1997) suggests that older adults with depression tend to score a little higher. It is copyrighted for commercial use and should be ordered from GL Assessment (http://shop.gl-assess-ment.co.uk/home.php?cat=417&gclid=CKaI7ZDI95cCFRNnQgodx23EDg).

The Patient Health Questionnaire (PHQ-9) (see Appendix) is widely used to screen for depression. It scores each of the nine DSM-IV criteria (Box 2.1) from '0' (not at all) to '3' (nearly every day). One or both of the first two questions should score at least '2' for depressive disorder to be likely. For a more definite diagnosis of major depression, five or more questions must be rated as 2 or 3, except for question 9, for which any score above '0' is significant. In addition, question 10, functional impairment, is endorsed as at least 'somewhat difficult'. Detailed information about scoring can be found at http://www.depression-primarycare.org/about/mission/.

The World Health Organization Well-Being Index was developed as a rapid screening test for depression. The 1998 version (version 2) is reproduced in the Appendix and has been validated on people aged 50 and above (Bonsignore *et al.* 2001). A higher score indicates greater well-being. A score below 13 or a score of 0 or 1 to any of the five items suggests a high likelihood of depressive disorder.

The Cornell Scale for detecting depression in dementia (Appendix) utilizes observational data and is administered to the patient's caregiver (Alexopoulos *et al.* 1988). It takes a little longer (15–20min) than the screening questionnaires but is more specific for depression in dementia than the other screening instruments.

Box 7.4 **Improving recognition of late-life depressive disorder**

- Remember that depressive disorder is not a normal part of ageing
- Maintain awareness of the high frequency of depressive disorders
- Become familiar with the core symptoms of depressive disorders
- And do not discount treatment because there seems to be an understandable cause
- And remember that the ageing process affects the presentation of depressive disorders
- Give equal attention to physical and metal health
- Develop skills for clinical interviewing of older persons
- Avoid therapeutic nihilism ('nothing works').

Given the importance of dementia as a differential diagnosis and a common co-morbidity, screening for dementia is important and for this the Mini-Mental State Examination (MMSE) is appropriate (Folstein *et al.* 1975). Its use is copyrighted (http://www.minimental.com/). Instructions for its use can be found on the UK Alzheimer's Society website (www.alzheimers.org.uk) following the links 'How Dementia is Diagnosed'. A shorter screening scale for dementia is the 6-item Orientation Memory-Concentration (OMC) test (Brooke and Bullock 2000).

Finally, the importance of improving practitioners' 'mindset' to increase detection cannot be overstated. Suggestions are given in Box 7.4. Some of these are linked to barriers to detection, discussed later in the chapter.

7.2 Depression severity

Also as part of the QoF primary care targets, in patients with a new diagnosis of depression there is a requirement to assess severity at the outset of treatment using an assessment tool validated for use in primary care (Quality Indicator DEP2). A new indicator for depression to reduce early cessation of treatment (DEP3) is being introduced based on the proportion of patients who have had a further assessment of severity 5–12 weeks after the first one. Box 7.5 lists three severity measures that are straightforward to use. Probably, the simplest is the PHQ that can also serve as a guide to treatment (Table 7.1).

The HDRS covers 17 items and is observer-rated (Hamilton 1960), whereas the MADRAS (Montgomery and Äsberg 1979) is a mixture of self-report and observed behaviour. If copied for any use other than individual research, the permission of the Royal College of Psychiatrists must be obtained. A 50% reduction in either scale is regarded as a treatment 'response' and a remission as a score of <7 or <10, respectively.

Box 7.5 Severity rating scales (see Appendix)
• PHQ
• 17-Item Hamilton Depression Rating Scale (HDRS)
• Montgomery–Åsberg Depression Rating Scale (MADRAS)

Table 7.1 Severity scales with the PHQ-9

PHQ-9 score	Provisional diagnosis	Treatment recommendation
5–9	Minimal symptoms	Support, educate to call if worse; return in 1 month
10–14	Minor depression	Support, watchful waiting
	Dysthymia	Antidepressant or psychotherapy
	Major depression, *mild*	Antidepressant or psychotherapy
15–19	Major depression, *moderately severe*	Antidepressant or psychotherapy
≥20	Major depression, *severe*	Antidepressant *and* psychotherapy (especially if not improved on monotherapy)

7.3 Suicide (see also Sections 3.2 and 8.4)

The risk factors for suicide are shown in Box 3.4. Suicide is sometimes viewed as a failure of specialist psychiatric services. In reality, most suicides involving older adults are not patients of psychiatric services and of those who do go on to end their lives, a majority have had contact with primary care services, so vigilance in primary care is vital for any preventive approach to be successful.

Primary care practitioners should take seriously statements concerning self-harm, attempt to remove a means of carrying out the act in those about whom they have concerns, and be alert to such behaviours such as suddenly altering wills, giving away possessions, or sudden changes in religious interest. Although they exist, over-reliance on suicide rating scales is unwise. The use of a relatively impersonal suicide rating questionnaire in someone who requires immense empathy might make matters worse. If in doubt, patients should undergo a specialist assessment.

7.4 Treatment principles

7.4.1 Deciding when to treat

There are concerns about medicalizing everyday problems in primary care, so the following three distinguishing characteristics are recommended to help come to a judgment about whether to treat depressive symptoms.

- *Duration*: symptoms are present for at least two weeks
- *Lack of fluctuation*: symptoms occur on most on most days, most of the time
- *Intensity*: of a degree that is definitely not normal for that individual and which interferes with function.

Figure 7.1 provides a framework for decision-making when making a diagnosis in primary care.

7.4.2 Deciding on treatment

Table 7.1, linked to the PHQ, provides a simple way to link severity to treatment modality. Table 7.2 takes this a little further, linking types of depression to particular treatment. It is especially important in primary care to consider an organic depressive disorder and to recognize psychotic depression. When treating older adults, GPs tend to select 'counselling' rather than the more evidence-based cognitive behavioural therapy (CBT) (Katona and Shankar 2004). This may be a resource issue but increasingly older people will expect a recognized psychological treatment.

7.4.3 Initiating treatment

Having decided what kind of depression is present and whether to initiate treatment, a framework is needed and this is shown in Table 6.1, the goals of treatment are as follows: risk reduction—of suicide or harm from self-neglect; remission of all depressive symptoms; to help the patient achieve optimal function; to treat the whole person, including somatic problems; and to prevent relapse and recurrence (discussed in Chapter 9). The patient's capacity and consent to treatment should always be checked (see Chapter 6, Section 6.3.3.1). Throughout treatment continue to educate the patient about depression and antidepressants and offer support.

For older patients inclined to attribute all symptoms to a somatic illness, time set aside to explain the nature and extent of any actual physical illness present and its likely effects is time well spent. Emphasizing that depression is an illness can help clinical engagement, as can explaining that it is common, treatable, and not a sign of moral weakness. Sometimes, it is too helpful to explore the ways in which both the patient and his or her family understand illness and its consequences in order to shed light on what might be the unconscious rewards of invalidism in patients who do not seem to be getting better. Patients must be encouraged to keep up as much activity and exercise as possible, perhaps keeping to a short 'programme' to encourage structure and purpose. Keeping to a balanced diet, avoiding over-eating and adhering to sleep hygiene are important. The latter includes avoiding caffeine drinks or alcohol at bed time and keeping to a regular pattern of returning to bed.

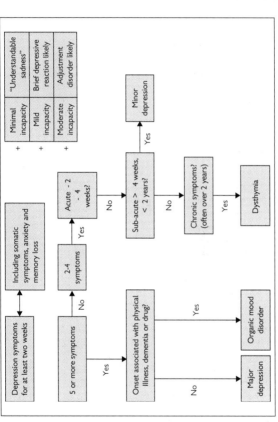

Figure 7.1 The differential diagnosis of depressive symptoms in later life

Table 7.2	
Type of depression	**Treatment modality**
Psychotic depression	Combined antidepressant and antipsychotic drugs; sometimes Electroconvulsive Therapy—urgent referral indicated
Organic depressive disorder	Treat underlying medical disorder/change offending medication May still have to treat depressive syndrome
Severe (non-psychotic depression)	Combined antidepressant and psychological therapy—consider referral
Mild–moderate depressive episode	Antidepressant or psychological therapy (CBT, problem-solving, IPT, or brief psychodynamic psychotherapy) either singly or in combination
Dysthymia	Antidepressant
Recent onset sub-threshold (minor) depression	Watchful waiting and support
Persistent sub-threshold (minor) depression	Antidepressant and support
Brief depression, grief reaction, and bereavement symptoms	Treat as for moderate depression if duration and intensity suggest intervention is indicated; otherwise, support and watchful waiting
Major depression with co-morbidity	Antidepressant and consider optimum analgesia where relevant
Persistent minor depression with co-morbidity	Some evidence of the effectiveness of counselling

Encouraging treatment concordance is vital as the most common reason for patients not getting better is that the treatment is not being taken properly or at all (Box 6.3). Patients often need reassurance that antidepressants are not addictive, and that depression is not 'senility' or a harbinger of dementia. They need to be warned not to expect immediate results. Commonly occurring side effects should be explained.

7.4.4 When to refer

In the United Kingdom, the process of depression management is guided by the stepped care process (NICE 2004) (Figure 7.2). Steps 1–3 are the domain of primary care. Knowing when to refer for specialist advice is important (Box 7.6) (Baldwin et al. 2003).

Who is responsible for care?	What is the focus?	What do they do?
Step 5: Inpatient care, crisis teams	Risk to life, severe self-neglect	Medication, combined treatments, ECT
Step 4: Mental health specialists including crisis teams	Treatment-resistant, recurrent, atypression, and psychotic depression, and those at significant risk	Medication, complex psychological interventions, combined treatments
Step 3: Primary care team, primary care mental health worker	Moderate or severe depression	Medication, psychological interventions, social support
Step 2: Primary care team, primary care mental health worker	Mild depression	Watchful waiting, guided self-help, computerised CBT, exercise, brief psychological interventions
Step 1: GP, practice nurse	Recognition	Assessment

Figure 7.2 NICE stepped care model of depression treatment.

7.4.5 **Supportive psychotherapy**

Offering support is not doing nothing. Combined with empathy and understanding it is a powerful therapeutic tool in depression, as is well known from the high placebo response rate in depression which is largely attributed to the effects of support.

7.5 **Barriers to treatment**

Barriers to accessing help for depression in primary care fall under the headings of patient-related, practitioner-related, organizational, and societal (Table 7.3). They especially disadvantage the elderly, poor, and minority populations who tend to have more ill health and are more disabled (Unützer et al. 1999). Ageism is a hidden barrier ('What's the point of treating depression at her age?'). No one sets out to be ageist but honest self-scrutiny is needed to guard against it.

7.6 **Collaborative care**

The collaborative care model has been developed to improve outcome in primary care. The components are a depression care manager (usually a nurse, psychologist, or social worker) who coordinates the care, including medication concordance supervised by a psychiatrist. Medication is provided by the GP. Regular review can occur by face-to-face interview or telephone contact. The 'IMPACT' study of older adults conducted in the United States is the largest to date (Unützer et al. 2002). A total of 1,801 depressed primary care patients (major depression, 17%; dysthymia, 30%; or both, 53%) were randomized to either usual care with active case management or usual care. There was a choice of Problem Solving Treatment (PST) or an antidepressant (prescribed by GP). At 12 months, 45% of intervention patients achieved a 50% reduction in symptoms compared with 19% of usual care subjects. Another large study from the United States, using a similar model, found some effect in reducing suicidal

Table 7.3 Barriers to consider in primary care

Factors	Possible barriers
Patient-related	• Somatization • Fear of stigmatization • Negative beliefs about antidepressant medication (e.g., that they are addictive) • False normalization of depression
Practitioner-related	• Poor consultation skills • Ageism • False normalization of depression • 'Therapeutic nihilism' • Attribution to societal ills • Lack of confidence and/or experience in treatments • Blinkered approach (seeing it as either physical or mental)
Organizational	• Separation of mental health and medical services • Poor co-ordination of services • Lack of appropriate services (e.g., psychological interventions) • Low reimbursement rates for psychotropic medication (in some countries)
Societal	• Lack of legislation regarding age discrimination

thinking (Bruce et al. 2004). In the United Kingdom, this model has also recently been shown to be effective (Chew-Graham et al. 2007). In addition, the use of a collaborative care approach to the management of residents in nursing homes who are depressed has been shown to improve outcomes (Llewellyn-Jones et al. 1999).

Simon et al. (2007) have provided evidence for the cost-effectiveness of the model as applied to patients with diabetes (not in old age) and the IMPACT study also found efficacy at modest cost.

7.7 Can depression be prevented? (see also Section 9.1)

Modelling has suggested substantial cost savings through the prevention of late-life depressive disorder (Smit et al. 2006). Risk factors are well known and include a prior history of depression, current depressive symptoms, chronic medical illness, vascular disease, functional limitation, female gender, insomnia, and a small social network (Cole and Dendukuri 2003). Other likely variables include genetic risk, early developmental difficulties, and dietary or metabolic factors. Some of these are modifiable. Prevention as a public health strategy is only realistic if there is a convenient way of detecting depression, a clear at-risk group, and an effective intervention. The two groups which might form a focus for the prevention of full-blown depressive disorder are those with prodromal symptoms (sub-threshold depression, Table 2.1) and those at risk, usually those with chronic handicapping illnesses, functional impairment, frequent contact with primary care, and a high level of home support.

Key references

Alexopoulos GS, Abrams RC, and Shamoian CA (1988). Cornell scale for depression in dementia. *Biological Psychiatry*, **23**(3), 271–84.

Baldwin R, Anderson D, Black S, et al. (2003). Guideline for the management of late-life depression in primary care. *International Journal of Geriatric Psychiatry*, **18**, 829–38.

Bonsignore M, Barkow K, Jessen F, and Heun R (2001). Validity of the five-item WHO Well-Being Index (WHO-5) in an elderly population. *European Archives of Psychiatry and Clinical Neuroscience*, **251**(Suppl. 2), II/27–II/31.

British Medical Association (BMA) (2006). Quality and outcomes framework guidance, p. 132. British Medical Association, London.

Brooke P and Bullock R (1999). Validation of the 6 item cognitive impairment test. *International Journal of Geriatric Psychiatry*, **14**, 936–40.

Bruce ML, Have TRT, Reynolds CF, et al. (2004). Reducing suicidal ideation and depressive symptoms in depressed older primary care patients: a randomized controlled trial. *JAMA*, **291**, 1081–91.

Chew-Graham CA, Lovell K, Roberts C, et al. (2007). Implementation of the Collaborative Care Model for the management of depression in the elderly in the UK. *British Journal of General Practice*, **57**, 364–70.

Cole MG and Dendukuri N (2003). Risk factors for depression among elderly community subjects. *The American Journal of Psychiatry*, **160**, 1147–56.

Folstein MF, Folstein SE, and McHugh PR (1975). "Mini-Mental State": a practical method for grading the cognitive state of patients for the clinician. *Journal of Psychiatric Research*, **12**, 185–98.

Hamilton M (1960). A rating scale for depression. *Journal of Neurology, Neurosurgery, and Psychiatry*, **23**, 56–62.

Iliffe S, Gould MM, and Mitchley S (1994). Evaluation of brief screening instruments for depression, dementia and problem drinking in general practice. *The British Journal of General Practice*, **44**, 503–7.

Katona CLE and Shankar KK (2004). Depression in old age. *Reviews in Clinical Gerontology*, **14**, 283–306.

Llewellyn-Jones RH, Baikie KA, Smithers H, Cohen J, Snowdon J, and Tennant CC (1999). Multifaceted shared care intervention for late life depression in residential care: randomised controlled trial. *BMJ*, **319**, 676–82.

Mitchell AJ and Coyne JC (2007). Do ultra-short screening instruments accurately detect depression in primary care: a pooled analysis and meta-analysis of 22 studies. *British Journal of General Practice*, **57**, 144–51.

Montgomery SA and Äsberg M (1979). A new depression scale designed to be sensitive to change. *British Journal of Psychiatry*, **134**, 382–9.

National Institute for Health and Clinical Excellence (NICE) (2004). Depression: management of depression in primary and secondary care—NICE guidance CG023. National Institute for Clinical Excellence, London.

Simon GE, Katon WJ, Lin EH, *et al.* (2007). Cost-effectiveness of systematic depression treatment among people with diabetes mellitus. *Archives of General Psychiatry*, **64**, 65–72.

Smit FR, Ederveen A, Cuijpers P, *et al.* (2006). Opportunities for cost-effective prevention of late-life depression. *Archives of General Psychiatry*, **63**, 290–6.

Spinhoven PH, Ormel J, Sloekers PPA, and Kempen G (1997). A validation study of the Hospital Anxiety and Depression Scale (HADS) in different groups of Dutch subjects. *Psychological Medicine*, **27**, 363–70.

Unützer J, Katon W, Sullivan M, and Miranda J (1999). Treating depressed older adults in primary care: narrowing the gap between efficacy and effectiveness. *The Millbank Quarterly*, **77**, 225–56.

Unützer J, Katon W, Callahan C, *et al.* (2002). Collaborative care management of late-life depression in the primary care setting. *JAMA*, **288**, 2836–45.

Zigmond AS and Snaith RP (1983). The hospital anxiety and depression scale. *Acta Psychiatrica Scandinavica*, **67**, 361–70.

Chapter 8

Prognosis

> **Key points**
> - Depression in later life is prone to recurrence.
> - Mortality may be increased in late-life depression.
> - Whether depression increases the rate of later dementia is controversial.

8.1 Outcome in naturalistic studies

In all age groups, depressive disorder is a condition prone to recurrence, which is why its management as a chronic (long-term) health condition makes sense. However, naturalistic studies (i.e., studies outside of controlled trials) provide evidence that under specialist care the prognosis is better than among those followed up in the community, where there may be great treatment variability or no treatment (Beekman *et al.* 2002). Why this is so is unclear but there are likely to be differences in risk factors, levels of detection, adequacy of treatment, and medical co-morbidity, all of which can influence outcome.

With regard to comparative outcome, Mitchell and Subramaniam (2005) reviewed the literature finding that episodes of depression remitted as well in later life as in other age groups, but there was a greater risk of relapse in older people. This was linked to two factors: age of onset (recurrent depression from earlier life associated with a poorer prognosis) and medical co-morbidity (associated with a later onset and worse prognosis). This suggests that interventions in the continuation and maintenance phases of treatment (Chapter 9) are especially important in late-life depression.

Compared to those without depression, patients who screen positive for depression whilst on a medical ward have a worse prognosis in terms of increased mortality and an increased likelihood of further care in a rehabilitation facility or a nursing home. In an acute hospital setting, an intervention package comprising problem-solving, brief support, and referral to relevant helping agencies did reduce depressive symptomatology but not length of stay (Baldwin *et al.* 2004).

8.2 Mortality

A number of studies suggest that having depression leads to an increased death rate in older adults. Blazer et al. (2001) though found that this effect was markedly attenuated if not abolished once factors such as chronic disease, health habits, cognitive impairment, functional impairment, and level social support were taken into account. This is still a controversial subject. Also controversial is the extent to which suicide contributes to an increase in mortality.

Several mechanisms to explain why depression may increase mortality in depressive disorders have been proposed (Box 8.1). These included the effects of co-morbid physical illness, occult illness (e.g., an unsuspected carcinoma), indirect effects of depression (e.g., pneumonia triggered by psychomotor retardation), treatment effects (e.g., some of the older tricyclic antidepressants are thought to be cardiotoxic), and biological effects (e.g., raised cortisol level). To these can be added behavioural factors (lack of exercise, smoking, alcohol misuse, poor diet, and limited activity), poorer health self-maintenance (e.g., never bothering to have blood pressure checked), and the consequences of the fact that depressed patients are less likely to adhere to medication for medical conditions.

Box 8.1 Possible mechanisms to explain increased mortality in depressive disorder

- Medical co-morbidity
- Illness effects (e.g., inertia from psychomotor retardation)
- Behavioural factors
  - Reduced physical activity
  - Poor diet
  - Smoking
  - Alcohol misuse
  - Poor health self-maintenance
- Poor adherence to prescribed medication
- Effects from occult illness (e.g., carcinoma not evident at diagnosis)
- Possible treatment effects (e.g., tricyclic drugs and cardiotoxicity)
- Biological factors (e.g., raised cortisol from chronic depression)

8.3 Prognostic factors

Predictive factors may be divided into *general factors* and those relevant to *characteristics of the* illness. Box 8.2 lists some of the poor outcome factors subdivided by illness features and general factors. Adversity includes chronic stress associated with a poor environment, crime and poverty, becoming a victim of crime, poor perceived social

Box 8.2 Poor outcome factors

Illness—clinical features
- Slower initial recovery
- More severe initial depression
- Duration more than 2 years
- Number of previous episodes (three and above increases risk)
- Chronic symptomatology with residual symptoms
- Psychotic depression
- Extensive disease of deep white matter and/or basal ganglia grey matter (vascular depression)
- Underlying organic brain disease (e.g., dementia)

General factors
- Chronic stress associated with poor environment, crime, and poverty
- A new physical illness
- Becoming a victim of crime
- Poor perceived (even if not objectively lacking) social support

support, and the development of serious physical ill health. Surprisingly, few features of the illness itself can be robustly linked with a poorer prognosis. The literature suggests that the following are important: a slow or incomplete recovery, three or more previous episodes, severity of initial depression, longer duration from onset (especially if over 2 years), and the presence of organic cerebral pathology.

8.4 Suicide (see also Sections 3.2 and 7.3)

In many countries where there are reliable data, suicide rates are highest among older adults. In the United States from 1980 to 1992, the suicide rate among those aged over 65 rose by 9% but among those aged 80–84 it increased by 35%. Some trends are surprising. For example, in a UK survey of the South Asian population, the highest rate was amongst women aged over 65 (McKenzie et al. 2008).

Suicide prevention programmes have been developed in a number of countries, often deploying a broad strategic approach with an emphasis on detection and treatment of depression. In Hong Kong, five suicide prevention teams aimed at older adults were established. These comprised psychiatrists, nurses, and social workers (Chiu et al. 2003). The teams work collaboratively with telephone support services, non-governmental organizations, centres for the elderly, and General Practitioners (GPs) to screen for depression and identify those at risk of suicide. Older people with suicidal risk or who are severely depressed are seen in fast-track clinics and visited at home by nurses, together with telephone monitoring. Another major focus is the provision of training for GPs in the detection and management of depression and collaborative care models of risk reduction (see Chapter 7).

There are factors that can reduce suicidal risk (Box 3.4). Given that pain and disability are associated with suicide, effective management of physical illness and control of pain may help to reduce this. In the United Kingdom, the suicide rate among elderly people fell after replacing coal gas with non-noxious natural gas, suggesting that removing a means of suicide may help prevention. Personal resilience is important—developing or regaining a sense of meaning and purpose in life is protective, as is religious practice.

8.5 **Dementia**

Whether depressive disorder predisposes to later dementia is a concern often raised by caregivers and patients. Sometimes, it is believed that depressive disorder in later life is the first sign of 'senility' (also Section 3.3). For those with normal cognition at the outset, reassurance can be given that developing dementia is no more likely than in anyone else. Follow-up data of patients with pseudodementia, however, show that they developed dementia at an increased rate. For this reason, it is important to conduct a brief cognitive screen at the outset. Patients with reversible cognitive impairment in the context of a depressive disorder should be followed up for signs of dementia. Evidence suggests that having recurrent depression severe enough to require hospitalization is associated with an increased risk of later dementia. Kessing & Andersen (2004) showed that the rate of dementia increased on average 13% (confidence interval 9% to 16%) with every episode leading to admission.

Key references

Baldwin R, Pratt H, Goring H, Marriott A, and Roberts C (2004). Does a nurse-led mental health liaison service for older people reduce psychiatric morbidity in acute general medical wards? A randomised controlled trial. *Age and Ageing*, **33**, 472–8.

Beekman AT, Geerlings SW, Deeg DJ, *et al.* (2002). The natural history of late-life depression. A 6-year prospective study in the community. *Archives of General Psychiatry*, **59**, 605–11.

Blazer D, Hybels C, and Pieper C (2001). The association of depression and mortality in elderly persons: a case for multiple independent pathways. *Journals of Gerontology Series A: Biological Sciences and Medical Sciences*, **56A**, M505–9.

Chiu HFK, Takahashi H, and Suh GH (2003). Elderly suicide prevention in East Asia. *International Journal of Geriatric Psychiatry*, **18**, 973–6.

Kessing LV, Anderson PK (2004). Does the risk of developing dementia increase with the number of episodes in patients with depressive disorder and in patients with bipolar disorder? *Journal of Neurology, Neurosurgery, and Psychiatry*, **75**, 1662–6.

McKenzie K, Bhui K, Nanchahal K, and Blizard B (2008). Suicide rates in people of South Asian origin in England and Wales: 1993–2003. *British Journal of Psychiatry*, **193**, 406–9.

Mitchell AJ and Subramaniam H (2005). Prognosis of depression in old age compared to middle age: a systematic review of comparative studies. *The American Journal of Psychiatry*, **162**, 1588–601.

Chapter 9

Prevention

Key points

- Primary prevention of late-life depression may be a realistic public health target.
- Secondary prevention is extremely effective.

The phases of depression treatment are illustrated in Figure 9.1 (Frank *et al.* 1991). The acute phase has already been covered. Continuation treatment follows remission and is aimed at preventing the return of symptoms (relapse). It is measured in months. Maintenance treatment aims to prevent future depressive episodes (recurrence) and is measured in years.

9.1 Primary prevention

Can depression be prevented? Risk factors already discussed (Section 7.7) include a family history of depression and a type of personality which limits the ability to make close relationships. In a meta-analysis of risk factors for late-life depression, Cole and Dendukuri (2003) highlighted five major risks: bereavement, sleep problems, physical disability, prior depression, and female gender. Some of these factors can be influenced via a public health preventative approach.

Figure 9.1 Conceptualization of phases of treatment in depression

Acute	Continuation	Maintenance
Via *response* To *remission* Weeks	Via *remission* To *recovery* About 12 months	Via *Recovery* To *prevent* *recurrence* Years

9.2 **Secondary prevention**

This refers to preventing future recurrences of depression or relapse soon after an episode. Continuation treatment typically lasts between 6 and 12 months, with old age psychiatrists tending to recommend the longer side of this interval. A pragmatic approach is to recommend a minimum of 12 months continuation treatment for a first episode, 24 months for a second, and at least 3 years for three or more episodes. In psychotic depression, antipsychotic medication is usually continued for 6 months with gradual withdrawal if the patient remains well.

Following recovery, there is considerable evidence that maintenance medication is effective in preventing a recurrence of depression. This has been demonstrated for tricyclic antidepressants, selective serotonin reuptake inhibitors (SSRIs), psychological treatments combined with antidepressants, lithium, and, more recently, atypical antipsychotics (Baldwin *et al.* 2003). As with other age groups, the general rule is to keep the antidepressant dose as close as possible to the one which the patient was taking on recovery ('the dose that got you well keeps you well').

Key references

Baldwin R, Anderson D, Black S, *et al.* (2003). Guideline for the management of late-life depression in primary care. *International Journal of Geriatric Psychiatry*, **18**, 829–38.

Cole MG and Dendukuri N (2003). Risk factors for elderly community subjects: a systematic review and meta-analysis. *American Journal of Psychiatry*, **160**, 1147–56.

Frank E, Prien RF, Jarrett RB, *et al.* (1991) Conceptualization and rationale for consensus definitions of terms in major depressive disorder. Remission, recovery, relapse, and recurrence. *Archives of General Psychiatry*, **48**(9), 851–5.

Chapter 10

Resources

There is a wealth of information to help patients, practitioners, and caregivers. The Internet in particular has led to an explosion of potential sources of help, although the quality cannot always be guaranteed. This chapter contains merely a fraction of what is available from reliable sources.

10.1 Practitioner resources

10.1.1 Treatment of depression

An Expert Consensus guideline from the United States led by Dr George Alexopoulos and colleagues has been published (Alexopoulos *et al.* 2001) and is outlined at http://www.psychguides.com/ (click on 'Available guidelines', then 'Depressive disorders in Older Patients'); the full guidance can be purchased from this link.

The Sections of Old Age Psychiatry and Affective Disorder of the World Health Organization have produced a guideline book for late-life depression (Baldwin *et al.* 2002). Google, with permission of the publisher, has sample chapters. Go to Google Book Search (http://books.google.com/) and type in Guidelines on Depression in Older People (you may need to register with Google).

A shorter guideline from the Faculty of Old Age Psychiatry of the UK Royal College of Psychiatrists (Baldwin *et al.* 2003) is available via the website of the *International Journal of Geriatric Psychiatry*. Those with journal access rights (e.g., Athens password) can download it.

Consensus Guidelines for Assessment and Management of Depression in the Elderly Faculty of Psychiatry of Old Age, NSW Branch, Royal Australian and New Zealand College of Psychiatrists is a short guide with a number of useful algorithms, including ones on assessment (including suicide risk evaluation) and treatment (http://www.health.nsw.gov.au/policy/cmh/publications/depression/depression_elderly.pdf) (alternatively go to the main New South Wales website and follow links from Centre for Mental Health).

The Canadian Coalition for Seniors' Mental Health (CCSMH) provides detailed guidelines on three relevant aspects: Assessment and Treatment of Depression; the Assessment and Treatment of Mental Health Issues in Long Term Care Homes (with a focus on mood and behavioural symptoms); and the Assessment of Suicide Risk and Prevention of Suicide. These are freely available (subject to registering on the website) by following the National Guideline Initiative link from the main website (http://www.ccsmh.ca/).

The British Association of Psychopharmacology (BAP) has a detailed evidence-based guideline on depression from the *Journal of Psychopharmacology* (Anderson *et al.* 2008) and accessible online at http://www.bap.org.uk/consensus/antidepressant.pdf.

In the United Kingdom, the National Institute of Health and Clinical Excellence (NICE) (http://www.nice.org.uk/) has a number of relevant guidelines. They include unipolar depression (NICE 2004b), bipolar disorder (NICE 2006b), electroconvulsive therapy (ECT) (NICE 2003), and self-harm (NICE 2004a).

Best treatment is a website which produces information from *British Medical Journal*'s Clinical Evidence (http://www.besttreatments.co.uk/btuk/conditions/1665.html). With the help of a mouse click, the viewer can see the evidence from the perspective of either patient or doctor.

10.1.2 Bipolar disorder

Although bipolar disorder is not a primary focus of this book, depression is a major cause of disability in patients with bipolar disorder. The BAP has published guidelines on Bipolar Disorder (Goodwin *et al.* 2003) which is accessible online (http://www.bap.org.uk/pdfs/FinalBipolarGuidelines.pdf). NICE (see Reference list) also has guidance which is again downloadable. The American Psychiatric Association (APA 2002) has a practice guideline from 2002 which is available to purchase from the APA website with an on-line update issued in 2005 (http://www.psych.org/psych_pract/treatg/pg/Bipolar.watch.pdf).

10.2 Patient education material

The **GDS** can be completed online via the GDS website (http://www.stanford.edu/~yesavage) (follow links to testing page).

The American Association for Geriatric Psychiatry has material on depression available through the website of The Geriatric Mental Health Foundation (GMHF): A Guide to Mental Wellness in Older Age: Recognizing and Overcoming Depression (A Depression Recovery Toolkit) and Depression in Late Life: Not a Natural Part of Aging (also available in Spanish) (http://www.gmhfonline.org/gmhf/consumer/index.html) or go to the GMHF website (http://www.gmhfonline.org) and follow links to Consumer/Patient information. The GMHF website also contains a number of useful links to other North American organizations.

Also from the United States, as part of the Expert Consensus Group led by George Alexopoulos and colleagues (above), a guide for patients and caregivers is available free at http://www.psychguides.com/ (click on 'Available guidelines', then 'Depressive disorders in Older Patients', and finally the guide).

The Healthy Minds, Healthy Lives initiative of the APA also has generic patient information leaflets (downloadable) for depression and bipolar disorder as part of its 'Let's Talk Facts' series (http://www.healthyminds.org/) (or go to the APA website and follow links to Public Information).

CANMAT (Canadian Network for Mood and Anxiety Treatments) is a not-for-profit research organization linking health care professionals from across Canada who have a special interest in mood and anxiety disorders. Its website mainly offers brief patient-oriented information about a range of common mental disorders, including depression in later life (http://www.canmat.org).

The Black Dog Institute is an educational, research, clinical, and community-oriented facility based in Australia dedicated to improving understanding, diagnosis, and treatment of mood disorders. It produces a number of fact sheets, including one on depression in old age (http://www.blackdoginstitute.org.au/factsheets/documents/DepressioninOlderPeople.pdf).

In the United Kingdom, the **Royal College of Psychiatrists** produces readable patient information, again including one on depression in later life (http://www.rcpsych.ac.uk/pdf/DOA.pdf).

See also MIND and Help the Aged (below).

10.3 Organizations for patients

The following sites are from the UK.

CRUSE Bereavement Centre
E-mail: helpline@crusebereavementcare.org.uk
Tel: 0870 167 1677

The Bipolar Organisation (formerly the Manic Depressive Fellowship)
Web: http://www.mdf.org.uk/
Tel: 08456 340 540 (UK Only); 0044 207 793 2600 (rest of the world)

MIND (National Association for Mental Health)
Mind, P.O. Box 277, Manchester M60 3XN
Web: http://www.mind.org.uk/
Tel: 0845 766 0163
Provides a variety of information including generic leaflets on depression, drugs to treat depression, and differentiating confusion, depression, and dementia. Information is available in Albanian, Arabic, Bengali, Chinese, Farsi, French, Gujarati, Hindi, Japanese, Punjabi, Somali, Spanish, Turkish, Urdu, and Welsh.

Depression Alliance

212 Spitfire Studios, 63-71 Collier Street, London N1 9BE

Web: www.depressionalliance.org

Tel: 0845 123 23 20

This provides information, support, and understanding to those who are affected by depression.

Help the Aged

207-221 Pentonville Road, London N1 9UZ

Web: http://www.helptheaged.org.uk/en-gb

Tel: 020 7278 1114; Fax: 020 7278 1116

Email: info@helptheaged.org.uk

The website has two downloadable leaflets entitled 'Beating the Blues' and 'Bereavement'.

Age Concern England

Astral House, 1268 London Road, London SW16 4ER

Web: http://www.ageconcern.org.uk/

Free telephone helpline: 0800 00 99 66

Campaigns on behalf of older people and provides factual information about commonly encountered difficulties.

Saneline

Web: www.sane.org.uk

Tel: 0845 767 8000

Saneline is a national out of hours telephone helpline providing information and support for anyone affected by mental health problems including families and carers.

There are numerous organisations around the world offering support. It is impossible to vouch for the accuracy of many of them and interested readers need to be aware that the Internet is not regulated. The following are reliable sites offering support for those with depression

DepNet is a Community on the Internet where people affected by depression and related diseases have the opportunity to meet and exchange experiences as well as finding information and help. DepNet is also a tool to support and help relatives. Countries offering local sites (with site language) include Argentina (Spanish), Australia (English), Brazil (Portuguese), Canada (English/French), Chile (Spanish), , Denmark (Danish), Estonia (Estonian), Greece (Greek), India (English), Korea (Korean), Malaysia (English), Mexico (Spanish), Pakistan (English), Philippines (English), Saudi Arabia (English/Arabic),

Singapore (English), South Africa (English), Turkey (Turkish), United Arab Emirates(English).
(http://www.depnet.com/)

The **Black Dog Institute** of Australia offers information about support groups in the territories of Australia
(http://www.blackdoginstitute.org.au/public/gettinghelp/supportgroups.cfm)

The **Canadian Network for Mood and Anxiety Treatments** gives information about support groups available in different Canadian States
(http://www.canmat.org/resources/findhelp.htm)

10.4 Self-help material

The British Association of Behavioural and Cognitive Psychotherapies (BABCP)
Globe Centre, P.O. Box 9, Accrington BB52GD, UK
Web: www.babcp.com
Tel: 01254 875277
The organization maintains a register of qualified practitioners and has a series of pamphlets (available for a small charge) covering anxiety, depression, insomnia, understanding CBT, and bipolar disorder to mention a few.

Oxford Cognitive Therapy Centre (OCTC)
Oxford Psychology Department, part of Oxfordshire Mental Healthcare NHS Trust, UK
Web: www.octc.co.uk
The website gives details of how to order a number of educational and self-help booklets with a CBT approach for a range of conditions including depression.

Self-help leaflets based on a CBT approach
This is written by members of the Newcastle, North Tyneside, and Northumberland Mental Health NHS Trust, England. This website has useful information and clear leaflets about common mental health issues including depression and bereavement.
Web: www.nnt.nhs.uk/mh/content.asp?PageName=selfhelp

Ultrasis
Web: www.ultrasis.com
Ultrasis produce interactive, computer-based CBT programmes for healthcare professionals, corporations, and consumers, including

Beating the Blues which has been endorsed for mild to moderate depression by the National Institute for Health and Clinical Excellence (NICE 2006a, technology assessment 97).

Key references

Alexopoulos GS, Katz IR, Reynolds CF, Carpenter D, and Docherty JP (2001). *The expert consensus guideline series: pharmacotherapy of depressive disorders in older patients.* Postgrad Med Special Report, pp. 1–86. Expert Knowledge Systems, L.L.C, McGraw-Hill Healthcare Information Programs, Minneapolis, MN.

American Psychiatric Association (APA) (2002). Practice guidelines for the treatment of patients with bipolar disorder. *American Journal of Psychiatry*, **159**(Suppl. 4), 1–50.

Anderson IM, Ferrier IN, Baldwin R, et al. (2008). On Behalf of the Consensus Meeting; endorsed by the British Association for Psychopharmacology—evidence-based guidelines for treating depressive disorders with antidepressants: a revision of the 2000 British Association for Psychopharmacology guidelines. *Journal of Psychopharmacology*, **22**, 343–96.

Baldwin RC, Chiu E, Katona C, and Graham N (2002). *Guidelines on depression in older people: practising the evidence.* Martin Dunitz, London, ISBN 1841841269.

Baldwin RC, Anderson D, Black S, et al. (2003). Faculty of Old Age Psychiatry Working Group, Royal College of Psychiatrists. Guideline for the management of late-life depression in primary care. *International Journal of Geriatric Psychiatry*, **18**(9), 829–38.

Goodwin GM, for the Consensus Group of the British Association for Psychopharmacology (2003). Evidence-based guidelines for treating bipolar disorder: recommendations from the British Association for Psychopharmacology. *Journal of Psychopharmacology*, 17, 149–73.

National Institute for Health and Clinical and Excellence (NICE) (2003). *The clinical effectiveness and cost effectiveness of electroconvulsive therapy (ECT) for depressive illness, schizophrenia, catatonia and mania TA 59.* National Institute for Clinical Excellence, London, April 2003.

National Institute for Health and Clinical and Excellence (NICE) (2004a). *Self-harm: the short-term physical and psychological management and secondary prevention of self-harm in primary and secondary care CG016.* National Institute for Clinical Excellence, London, July 2004.

National Institute for Health and Clinical Excellence (NICE) (2004b). *Depression: management of depression in primary and secondary care— NICE guidance CG023.* National Institute for Clinical Excellence, London, December 2004.

National Institute for Health and Clinical Excellence (NICE) (2006a). *Depression and anxiety—computerised cognitive behavioural therapy (CCBT). Health Technology Assessment No 97.* National Institute for Clinical Excellence, London, February 2006.

National Institute for Health and Clinical Excellence (NICE) (2006b). *Bipolar disorder: the management of bipolar disorder in adults, children and adolescents, in primary and secondary care. NICE clinical guideline 38*. National Institute for Clinical Excellence, London, July 2006.

General reading

Alexopoulos GS (2005). Depression in the elderly. *The Lancet*, **365**(9475), 1961–70.

Baldwin RC, Chiu E, Katona C, and Graham N (2002). *Guidelines on depression in older people: practising the evidence under the auspices of the World Psychiatric Association Sections of Old Age Psychiatry and Affective Disorders*. Martin Dunitz, London.

Blazer DG (2003). Depression in late life: review and commentary. *Journal of Gerontology: Medical Sciences*, **58A**, 249–65.

Katona CLE and Shankar KK (2004). Depression in old age. *Reviews in Clinical Gerontology*, **14**, 283–306.

Taylor D, Paton C, and Kerwin R (2007). *The Maudsley prescribing guidelines*, 9th edn. Informa Health care, London.

Unützer J (2007). Late-life depression. *New England Journal of Medicine*, **357**, 2269–76.

WPA/PTD Educational Program on Depressive Disorders. Module 1: overview and fundamental aspects. Module 3: depressive disorders in older persons. Available online at: http://www.wpanet.org/education/ed-program-guidelines.shtml.

Appendix

Sample rating scales

Table A.1 Sample rating scales used in the assessment of depression in later life

Rating scale	Key features	Administrator	Time taken (min)
Geriatric Depression Scale (GDS)	Available in 30-, 15-, and 4-item versions; easy to administer; available online; many translations	Patient or patient-assisted	10
Patient Health Questionnaire (PHQ-9)	Uses criteria from DSM-IV (Box 2.1); brief and useful as primary care screen	Patient	5
The World Health Organization Well-Being Index	Only five questions; brief primary care screen; scoring a little complicated; validated in older people	Patient	5
Cornell Scale for Depression in Dementia	Only validated scale for depression in dementia; takes more time than a screening questionnaire	Clinician via carers or other observers	15–20
Hamilton Depression Rating Scale (HDRS)	Widely used in clinical trials; requires knowledge of mental health; perhaps overly focussed on somatic symptoms	Clinician	15
Montgomery and Åsberg Depression Rating Scale (MADRAS)	Widely used in clinical trials; non-specialist; sensitive to change	Clinician	15

A.1 **Geriatric Depression Scale (GDS)**

Table A.2 Sample rating sheet from the GDS

Instructions: Choose the best answer for how you have felt over the past <u>week</u>.

   1. Are you basically satisfied with your life? No
   2. Have you dropped many of your activities and interests? Yes
   3. Do you feel your life is empty? Yes
   4. Do you often get bored? Yes
   5. Are you hopeful about the future? No
   6. Are you bothered by thoughts you can't get out of your head? Yes
   7. Are you in good spirits most of the time? No
   8. Are you afraid something bad is going to happen to you? Yes
   9. Do you feel happy most of the time? No
   10. Do you often feel helpless? Yes
   11. Do you often get restless and fidgety? Yes
   12. Do you prefer to stay at home, rather than going out and doing new things? Yes
   13. Do you frequently worry about the future? Yes
   14. Do you feel you have more problems with your memory than most? Yes
   15. Do you think it is wonderful to be alive now? No
   16. Do you often feel down-hearted and blue (sad)? Yes
   17. Do you feel pretty worthless the way you are? Yes
   18. Do you worry a lot about the past? Yes
   19. Do you find life very exciting? No
   20. Is it hard for you to start on new projects (plans)? Yes
   21. Do you feel full of energy? No
   22. Do you feel that your situation is hopeless? Yes
   23. Do you think most people are better off (in their lives) than you are? Yes
   24. Do you frequently get upset over little things? Yes
   25. Do you frequently feel like crying? Yes
   26. Do you have trouble concentrating? Yes
   27. Do you enjoy getting up in the morning? No
   28. Do you prefer to avoid social gatherings (get-togethers)? Yes
   29. Is it easy for you to make decisions? No
   30. Is your mind as clear as it used to be? No

Note: (1) Answers refer to responses which score '1'; (2) bracketed phrases refer to alternative ways of expressing the questions; (3) questions in bold comprise the 15-item version.

Suggested meaning of scores (GDS30):

0–4: normal, depending on age, education, complaints; 5–8: mild; 8–11: moderate; 12–15: severe; and thresholds for possible 'case' of depression ≥5 for GDS15 and ≥2 for GDS4.

A.2 The Patient Health Questionnaire (PHQ-9)

Name:_____ Date:_____

Over the past 2 weeks, how often have you been bothered by any of the following problems? (use "✓" to indicate your answer)

	Not at all	Several days	More than half the days	Nearly every day
1. Little interest or pleasure in doing things	0	1	2	3
2. Feeling down, depressed, or hopeless	0	1	2	3
3. Trouble falling or staying asleep, or sleeping too much	0	1	2	3
4. Feeling tired or having little energy	0	1	2	3
5. Poor appetite or overeating	0	1	2	3
6. Feeling bad about yourself— or that you are a failure or have let yourself or your family down	0	1	2	3
7. Trouble concentrating on things, such as reading the newspaper or watching television	0	1	2	3
8. Moving or speaking so slowly that other people could have noticed. Or the opposite— being so fidgety or restless that you have been moving around a lot more than usual	0	1	2	3
9. Thoughts that you would be better off dead, or of hurting yourself in some way	0	1	2	3
	add columns		+	+
(Healthcare professional: For interpretation of TOTAL, please refer to accompanying scoring card.)	**Total:**			
10. If you checked off any problems, how difficult have these problems made it for you to do your work, take care of things at home, or get along with other people?	Not difficult at all _____ Somewhat difficult _____ Very difficult _____ Extremely difficult _____			

A.3 The World Health Organization Well-Being Index

	Over the last two weeks	All of the time	Most of the time	More than half of the time	Less than half of the time	Some of the time	At no time
1	I have felt cheerful and in good spirits	❏ 5	❏ 4	❏ 3	❏ 2	❏ 1	❏ 0
2	I have felt calm and relaxed	❏ 5	❏ 4	❏ 3	❏ 2	❏ 1	❏ 0
3	I have felt active and vigorous	❏ 5	❏ 4	❏ 3	❏ 2	❏ 1	❏ 0
4	I woke up feeling fresh and rested	❏ 5	❏ 4	❏ 3	❏ 2	❏ 1	❏ 0
5	My daily life has been filled with things that interest me	❏ 5	❏ 4	❏ 3	❏ 2	❏ 1	❏ 0

A.4 Hamilton Rating Scale for Depression

1 DEPRESSED MOOD (sadness, hopeless, helpless, worthless)

0   ❏ Absent.
1   ❏ These feeling states indicated only on questioning.
2   ❏ These feeling states spontaneously reported verbally.
3   ❏ Communicates feeling states non-verbally, i.e. through facial expression, posture, voice and tendency to weep.
4   ❏ Patient reports virtually only these feeling states in his/her spontaneous verbal and non-verbal communication.

2 FEELINGS OF GUILT

0   ❏ Absent.
1   ❏ Self-reproach, feels he/she has let people down.
2   ❏ Ideas of guilt or rumination over past errors or sinful deeds.
3   ❏ Present illness is a punishment. Delusions of guilt.
4   ❏ Hears accusatory or denunciatory voices and/or experiences threatening visual hallucinations.

3 SUICIDE

0   ❏ Absent.
1   ❏ Feels life is not worth living.
2   ❏ Wishes he/she were dead or any thoughts of possible death to self.
3   ❏ Ideas or gestures of suicide.
4   ❏ Attempts at suicide (any serious attempt rate 4).

4 INSOMNIA: EARLY IN THE NIGHT

0   ❏ No difficulty falling asleep.
1   ❏ Complains of occasional difficulty falling asleep, i.e. more than 1/2 hour.
2   ❏ Complains of nightly difficulty falling asleep.

5 INSOMNIA: MIDDLE OF THE NIGHT

0 ❏ No difficulty.

1 ❏ Patient complains of being restless and disturbed during the night.

2 ❏ Waking during the night—any getting out of bed rates 2 (except for purposes of voiding).

6 INSOMNIA: EARLY HOURS OF THE MORNING

0 ❏ No difficulty.

1 ❏ Waking in early hours of the morning but goes back to sleep.

2 ❏ Unable to fall asleep again if he/she gets out of bed.

7 WORK AND ACTIVITIES

0 ❏ No difficulty.

1 ❏ Thoughts and feelings of incapacity, fatigue or weakness related to activities, work or hobbies.

2 ❏ Loss of interest in activity, hobbies or work—either directly reported by the patient or indirect in listlessness, indecision and vacillation (feels he/she has to push self to work or activities).

3 ❏ Decrease in actual time spent in activities or decrease in productivity. Rate 3 if the patient does not spend at least three hours a day in activities (job or hobbies) excluding routine chores.

4 ❏ Stopped working because of present illness. Rate 4 if patient engages in no activities except routine chores, or if patient fails to perform routine chores unassisted.

8 RETARDATION (slowness of thought and speech, impaired ability to concentrate, decreased motor activity)

0 ❏ Normal speech and thought.

1 ❏ Slight retardation during the interview.

2 ❏ Obvious retardation during the interview.

3 ❏ Interview difficult.

4 ❏ Complete stupor.

9 AGITATION

0 ❏ None.

1 ❏ Fidgetiness.

2 ❏ Playing with hands, hair, etc.

3 ❏ Moving about, can't sit still.

4 ❏ Hand wringing, nail biting, hair-pulling, biting of lips.

10 ANXIETY PSYCHIC

0 ❏ No difficulty.

1 ❏ Subjective tension and irritability.

2 ❏ Worrying about minor matters.

3 ❏ Apprehensive attitude apparent in face or speech.

4 ❏ Fears expressed without questioning.

11 ANXIETY SOMATIC (physiological concomitants of anxiety) such as:
gastro-intestinal—dry mouth, wind, indigestion, diarrhea, cramps, belching; cardiovascular—palpitations, headaches; respiratory—hyperventilation, sighing, urinary frequency, sweating

0 ❏ Absent.

1 ❏ Mild.

2 ❏ Moderate.

3 ❏ Severe.

4 ❏ Incapacitating.

12 SOMATIC SYMPTOMS GASTRO-INTESTINAL

0 ❏ None.

1 ❏ Loss of appetite but eating without staff encouragement. Heavy feelings in abdomen.

2 ❏ Difficulty eating without staff urging. Requests or requires laxatives or medication for bowels or medication for gastro-intestinal symptoms.

13 GENERAL SOMATIC SYMPTOMS

0 ❏ None.

1 ❏ Heaviness in limbs, back or head. Backaches, headaches, muscle aches. Loss of energy and fatigability.

2 ❏ Any clear-cut symptom rates 2.

14 GENITAL SYMPTOMS (symptoms such as loss of libido, menstrual disturbances)

0 ❏ Absent.

1 ❏ Mild.

2 ❏ Severe.

15 HYPOCHONDRIASIS

0 ❏ Not present.

1 ❏ Self-absorption (bodily).

2 ❏ Preoccupation with health.

3 ❏ Frequent complaints, requests for help, etc.

4 ❏ Hypochondriacal delusions.

16 LOSS OF WEIGHT (RATE EITHER a OR b)

(a) According to the patient:

0 ❏ No weight loss

1 ❏ Probable weight loss associated with present illness in week

2 ❏ Definite (according to patient) weight loss

(b) According to weekly measurements:

0 ❏ Less than 1 lb in week.

1 ❏ Greater than 1 lb weight loss in week.

2 ❏ Greater than 2 lb weight loss in week.

17 INSIGHT

0 ❑ Acknowledges being depressed and ill.

1 ❑ Acknowledges illness but attributes cause to bad food, climate, overwork, virus, need for rest, etc.

2 ❑ Denies being ill at all.

Total score: _____

A.5 **Montgomery and Äsberg Depression Rating Scale**

1. Apparent sadness

Representing despondency, gloom and despair (more than just ordinary transient low spirits), reflected in speech, facial expression, and posture. Rate by depth and inability to brighten up.

0 = No sadness. ❏

2 = Looks dispirited but does brighten up without difficulty. ❏

4 = Appears sad and unhappy most of the time. ❏

6 = Looks miserable all the time. Extremely despondent. ❏

2. Reported sadness

Representing reports of depressed mood, regardless of whether it is reflected in appearance or not.

Includes low spirits, despondency or the feeling of being beyond help and without hope.

0 = Occasional sadness in keeping with the circumstances. ❏

2 = Sad or low but brightens up without difficulty. ❏

4 = Pervasive feelings of sadness or gloominess. The mood is still influenced by external circumstances. ❏

6 = Continuous or unvarying sadness, misery or despondency. ❏

3. Inner tension

Representing feelings or ill-defined discomfort, edginess, inner turmoil, mental tension mounting to either panic, dread or anguish. Rate according to intensity, frequency, duration and the extent of reassurance called for.

0 = Placid. Only fleeting inner tension. ❏

2 = Occasional feelings of edginess and ill-defined discomfort. ❏

4 = Continuous feelings of inner tension or intermittent panic which the patient can only master with some difficulty. ❏

6 = Unrelenting dread or anguish. Overwhelming panic. ❏

4. Reduced sleep

Representing the experience of reduced duration or depth of sleep compared to the subject's own normal pattern when well.

0 = Sleeps as usual. ❏

2 = Slight difficulty dropping off to sleep or slightly reduced, ❏
light or fitful sleep.

4 = Sleep reduced or broken by at least 2 hours. ❏

6 = Less than 2 or 3 hours sleep. ❏

5. Reduced appetite

Representing the feeling of a loss of appetite compared with when well. Rate by loss of desire for food or the need to force oneself to eat.

0 = Normal or increased appetite. ❏

2 = Slightly reduced appetite. ❏

4 = No appetite. Food is tasteless. ❏

6 = Needs persuasion to eat at all. ❏

6. Concentration difficulties

Representing difficulties in collecting one's thoughts mounting to an incapacitating lack of concentration. Rate according to intensity, frequency, and degree of incapacity produced.

0 = No difficulties in concentrating. ❏

2 = Occasional difficulties in collecting one's thoughts. ❏

4 = Difficulties in concentrating and sustaining thought which ❏
reduces ability to read or hold a conversation.

6 = Unable to read or converse without great difficulty. ❏

7. Lassitude

Representing difficulty in getting started or slowness in initiating and performing everyday activities.

0 = Hardly any difficulty in getting started. No sluggishness. ❏

2 = Difficulties in starting activities. ❏

4 = Difficulties in starting simple routine activities, which are ❏
carried out with effort.

6 = Complete lassitude. Unable to do anything without help. ❏

8. Inability to feel

Representing the subjective experience of reduced interest in the surroundings, or activities that normally give pleasure. The ability to react with adequate emotion to circumstances or people is reduced.

0 = Normal interest in the surroundings and in other people.   ❏

2 = Reduced ability to enjoy usual interests.   ❏

4 = Loss of interest in the surroundings. Loss of feelings for friends and acquaintances.   ❏

6 = The experience of being emotionally paralysed, inability to feel anger, grief or pleasure and a complete or even painful failure to feel for close relatives and friends.   ❏

9. Pessimistic thoughts

Representing thoughts of guilt, inferiority, self-reproach, sinfulness, remorse and ruin.

0 = No pessimistic thoughts.   ❏

2 = Fluctuating ideas of failure, self-reproach or self-depreciation.   ❏

4 = Persistent self-accusation, or definite but still rational ideas of guilt or sin. Increasingly pessimistic about the future.   ❏

6 = Delusions of ruin, remorse or irredeemable sin. Self-accusations, which are absurd and unshakable.   ❏

10. Suicidal thoughts

Representing the feeling that life is not worth living, that a natural death would be welcome, suicidal thoughts, and preparations for suicide. Suicide attempts should not in themselves influence the rating.

0 = Enjoys life or takes it as it comes.   ❏

2 = Weary of life. Only fleeting suicidal thoughts.   ❏

4 = Probably better off dead. Suicidal thoughts are common, and suicide is considered as a possible solution, but without specific plans or intent.   ❏

6 = Explicit plans for suicide when there is an opportunity. Active preparations for suicide.   ❏

Reproduced from BJP, **134**, 382–389, with the permission of the Royal College of Psychiatrists.

A.6 Cornell Scale for Depression in Dementia

Patient status: ❏ Nursing Home Resident ❏ Outpatient   ❏ Inpatient

Informant used: ❏ Yes   ❏ No

Scores: 0 = absent   1 = mild or   2 = severe   9999 = unable to
                              intermittent   evaluate

Ratings should be based on symptoms and signs occurring during the week prior to interview.

If severe and intermittent, score as severe. No score should be given if symptoms result from physical disability or illness.

APPENDIX **Sample rating scales**

	INFORMANT			PATIENT			RATER'S OPINION		
A. MOOD RELATED SIGNS										
1. ANXIETY	0	1	2	9999	0	1	2	9999	0	1	2	9999
Anxious expression, ruminations, worrying										
2. SADNESS	0	1	2	9999	0	1	2	9999	0	1	2	9999
Sad expression, sad voice, tearfulness										
3. LACK OF REACTIVITY TO PLEASANT EVENTS	0	1	2	9999	0	1	2	9999	0	1	2	9999
4. IRRITABILITY	0	1	2	9999	0	1	2	9999	0	1	2	9999
Easily annoyed, short tempered										
B. BEHAVIORAL DISTURBANCE										
5. AGITATION	0	1	2	9999	0	1	2	9999	0	1	2	9999
Restlessness, handwringing, hairpulling										
6. RETARDATION	0	1	2	9999	0	1	2	9999	0	1	2	9999
Slow movements, slow speech, slow reactions										
7. MULTIPLE PHYSICAL COMPLAINTS	0	1	2	9999	0	1	2	9999	0	1	2	9999
(score 0 if GI symptoms only)										
8. LOSS OF INTEREST	0	1	2	9999	0	1	2	9999	0	1	2	9999
Less involved in usual activities (score only if change occurred acutely i.e.: in less than 1 month)										

C. PHYSICAL SIGNS

9. APPETITE LOSS Eating less than usual	0	1	2	9999	0	1	2	9999
10. WEIGHT LOSS (score 2 if greater than 5 lbs. in 1 month)	0	1	2	9999	0	1	2	9999
11. LACK OF ENERGY Fatigues easily, unable to sustain activities (score only if change occurred acutely i.e.: in less than 1 month)	0	1	2	9999	0	1	2	9999

D. CYCLIC FUNCTIONS

12. DIURNAL VARIATION OF MOOD Symptoms worse in the morning	0	1	2	9999	0	1	2	9999
13. DIFFICULTY FALLING ASLEEP Later than usual for this individual	0	1	2	9999	0	1	2	9999
14. MULTIPLE AWAKENINGS DURING SLEEP	0	1	2	9999	0	1	2	9999
15. EARLY MORNING AWAKENINGS Earlier than usual for this individual	0	1	2	9999	0	1	2	9999

	INFORMANT			PATIENT			RATER'S OPINION		
E. IDEATIONAL DISTURBANCE									
16. SUICIDE Feels life is not worth living, has suicidal wishes, or make suicide attempt	0	1	2	9999	0	1	2	9999	0	1	2	9999
17. SELF-DEPRECIATION Self-blame, poor self esteem, feelings of failure	0	1	2	9999	0	1	2	9999	0	1	2	9999
18. PESSIMISM Anticipation of the worst	0	1	2	9999	0	1	2	9999	0	1	2	9999
19. MOOD CONGRUENT DELUSIONS Delusions of poverty, illness, or loss	0	1	2	9999	0	1	2	9999	0	1	2	9999

Reproduced from Biological Psychiatry, 23/3, Alexopoulos GS et al., Cornell scale for depression in dementia, 14, © 1988, with permission from Elsevier.

Key references

Alexopoulos GS, Abrams RC, and Shamoian CA (1988). Cornell Scale for Depression in Dementia. *Biological Psychiatry*, **23**(3), 271–84.

Bonsignore M, Barkow K, Jessen F, and Heun R (2001). Validity of the five-item WHO Well-Being Index (WHO-5) in an elderly population. *European Archives of Psychiatry and Clinical Neuroscience*, **251**(Suppl. 2), II/27–II/31.

Hamilton M (1960). A rating scale for depression. *Journal of Neurology, Neurosurgery, and Psychiatry*, **23**, 56–62.

Montgomery SA and Äsberg M (1979). A new depression scale designed to be sensitive to change. *British Journal of Psychiatry*, **134**, 382–9.

Index